HEALTH POLICY IN THE UNITED STATES
Access, Cost and Quality

B. Guy Peters

First published in Great Britain in 2024 by

Policy Press, an imprint of
Bristol University Press
University of Bristol
1–9 Old Park Hill
Bristol
BS2 8BB
UK
t: +44 (0)117 374 6645
e: bup-info@bristol.ac.uk

Details of international sales and distribution partners are available at policy.bristoluniversitypress.co.uk

British Library Cataloguing in Publication Data
A catalogue record for this book is available from the British Library

ISBN 978-1-4473-5775-9 hardcover
ISBN 978-1-4473-5776-6 paperback
ISBN 978-1-4473-5777-3 ePub
ISBN 978-1-4473-5778-0 ePdf

Cover design: Nicky Borowiec
Front cover image: Adobe Stock/Stefano Garau

Contents

List of tables and boxes

Tables

Boxes

Preface

This book has been a very long time in the making. I began to be interested in health policy in the early 1970s when at the University of Delaware. I taught a class on the social and political dimensions of health with an anthropologist and a sociologist, both of whom, unlike me, were experts in the field. This learning experience was followed by another at the School of Public Health and Tropical Medicine at Tulane University, working with a friend who also was much more of a specialist than I was.

When I arrived at the University of Pittsburgh in 1984, I found that I had a colleague who was already teaching health policy very well, so I continued teaching and writing about public policy more generally until he retired. The interest in health policy had remained alive, but it had to simmer for a while on the back burner. Once I began teaching health policy at Pitt, my interest grew even more and, after a half dozen iterations of the course, I think I have acquired enough information and sufficient perspective on the field to be able to write a book that covers the field, at least to a certain depth.

This book does attempt to cover the field and to discuss the most important topics in health policy. This is an extremely complex field of public policy—most are, but this seems even more complex—and therefore one book cannot go into every detail. What I have attempted to do is to highlight the three big questions—access, cost and quality. I have also attempted to demonstrate that several perspectives, such as the jungle concept, can help to understand the difficulties faced by patients in dealing with the healthcare system, and also some of the general dysfunctions of that system. Those problems have political consequences, and those too are central to the analysis in the book.

Without being aware of it, the students in the six iterations of this course have helped me to develop the book. They have asked good questions—those to which I did not initially know the answers—and have written interesting papers that illuminated some aspect or another of the US healthcare system. More directly, Lauren Wright, who has worked as my undergraduate research assistant for the past 18 months, has been an extremely valuable contributor to the project. And I should also mention my colleague and friend Bert Rockman, who shares my interest and with whom I have had numerous interesting discussions.

In addition to informing readers about US health policy I hope the book may also produce some action. As good as healthcare can be here, it is also highly unequal, too expensive and, at times, careless. I hope this recounting of the issues will be one more push in the direction of change.

B. Guy Peters
Verona, PA

1

Introduction: Images of American healthcare

All people depend upon healthcare of some form or another. This healthcare may be traditional medicine given by a healer in a village, or it may be high-tech medicine delivered in a massive modern hospital, or something in between. Whatever the level of technology or the underlying model of medicine and health in question (see for example Leslie, 1976) people want to have some way of coping with disease, or perhaps the realities of aging. Americans are certainly no different, and indeed may be more dependent upon medical interventions than most other cultures (Stein, 2018).

Healthcare in the United States is a huge industry that has a major impact on the society and the economy. The centrality of healthcare has become even more evident during the crisis caused by the coronavirus, and the crucial role that the medical industry played in American life from spring 2020 onward. Healthcare providers were hailed as heroes during this time, at the same time that some politicians and bloggers denied the existence of the disease, or the efficacy of the vaccines. Despite that centrality, the health sector in the United States does, however, have a number of paradoxical elements. The most obvious and important of these paradoxes is that although spending on healthcare is the highest in the world as a percentage of gross domestic product (GDP), health outcomes are not as good as in many other countries that spend much less.

The magnitude of spending for healthcare is shown in Table 1.1. More than one dollar in six in the American economy is spent on healthcare in some form or another. This rate of expenditure is higher than any other consolidated democracy. If we consider that the per capita GDP of the United States is higher than that of most other countries then the per capita spending on healthcare is even more out of line with other countries. The differences in spending are even greater when the higher GDP of the United States is considered. Per capita spending is almost 70 percent greater in the US than in the second highest spending country, Switzerland. Healthcare is important and even in the more frugal countries, such as the United Kingdom, included in Table 1.1, it represents a significant share of the national economy; but the United States stands out in just how much is spent. Therefore, two of the principal questions in this book will be why is healthcare so expensive, and what can be done about reducing expenditures.

At the same time that American healthcare is very expensive it is not as effective as it might be, and outcomes for American citizens are not as good as they are in many other countries. If we look at two standard measures of healthcare quality—infant mortality and life expectancy—the United States does not compare well

Table 1.1: Healthcare expenditures of the United States in comparative perspective, 2019

A. Spending as a Percentage of GDP	
United States	16.8
Germany	11.7
Switzerland	11.3
France	11.1
Japan	11.0
Sweden	10.9
Canada	10.8
United Kingdom	10.2
Netherlands	10.2
New Zealand	9.1
Iceland	8.7
B. Per Capita Spending ($US, converted with Purchasing Power Parities)	
United States	11,945
Switzerland	7,138
Germany	6,731
Netherlands	6,299
Sweden	5,754
France	5,564
Canada	5,370
United Kingdom	5,268
Japan	4,691
Comparable Country Average	5,736

Source: Wager et al. (2022).

with other wealthy countries, or even to some less wealthy countries. Tables 1.2 and 1.3 shows the ranking of the United States on those two variables, along with a sampling of other countries. The performance of the United States is poorer than a number of other countries, almost all of which are poorer than the United States. Further, infant mortality for Black babies in the United States is 10.6 per 1,000 live births, a figure similar to El Salvador.

It is important at this juncture to point out that health outcomes are not entirely a function of the quality of the healthcare system. Given the amount of money spent directly on health, these outcomes do not appear positive. However, these poor outcomes also reflect high levels of income inequality in the United States, and high levels of inequality in access to health facilities and professionals. That inequality is defined by region, income, race and a number of other factors.

Table 1.2: Infant mortality rates, 2022,[1] number and rank

Iceland	1.54 (1)
Estonia	1.65 (3)
Slovenia	1.76 (4)
Norway	1.79 (5)
Japan	1.82 (6)
Singapore	1.85 (7)
Finland	1.88 (8)
Montenegro	1.95 (9)
Sweden	2.15 (10)
Belarus	2.19 (11)
Italy	2.47 (17)
Spain	2.71 (21)
Germany	3.1 (25)
France	3.45 (31)
United Kingdom	3.62 (35)
Cuba	4.08 (39)
Uruguay	5.32 (48)
United States	5.44 (50)
China	5.47 (51)
Lebanon	5.97 (59)
Thailand	7.41 (66)
Peru	9.95 (77)
Mexico	11.77 (87)
Brazil	13.13 (97)
Philippines	20.95 (123)
Haiti	46.66 (172)
Sierra Leone	80.1 (195)

[1] Deaths in the first year of life per 1,000 live births.
Source: World Health Organization, Global Health Observatory.

Further, these poor outcomes reflect the amount of gun violence in the country, with almost 50,000 people being killed by guns in 2021.[1]

The pandemic of a novel coronavirus also raised questions about the quality of American medical care. The weaknesses in public health, especially in testing and contact tracing, were very apparent, and might be more expected in a medical care system oriented toward private practice and curative medicine (Hicks and Biddinger, 2020). But the death rate of infected patients was one of the highest in the world. These numbers might be explained in part by the lower levels of testing

Table 1.3: Female life expectancy at birth, 2021

Japan	87.8
South Korea	87.1
France	86.0
Italy	86.0
Switzerland	85.9
Australia	85.5
Sweden	85.1
Canada	84.8
Israel	84.5
United Kingdom	83.8
Germany	83.4
Chile	81.8
China	81.3
United States	81.0
Poland	80.8
Mexico	78.2
Chad	54.7

Source: United Nations, main database, https://data.un.org/Data.aspx?q=life+expectancy&d=PopDiv&f=variableID%3A67.

in the United States, so that asymptomatic cases were not a part of the denominator. And it could also be explained in part by the prevalence of co-morbidities such as heart disease, asthma and obesity among the fatal cases. But these mitigating factors do not totally explain the poor showing of the healthcare system.

In addition to the relatively poor performance on indicators of the quality of health services, even given all the money spent a significant number of the American population does not have access to health insurance or other means of receiving healthcare. Even after the adoption of the Affordable Care Act and its associated expansion of Medicaid, there are approximately 30 million Americans who lack health insurance, and millions more who have inadequate health insurance (PGPF, 2022).

A second paradox in American healthcare is that, despite the rather mediocre outcomes in total, some of the most advanced research and healthcare provision in the world is found in the United States. The United States spends far more on healthcare research than any other country. For many Americans healthcare is almost unattainable, while for many it is readily available, with insurance provided by their employer, These differences among different segments of the population help to account for the first paradox. The high levels of expenditure for the better insured and more affluent citizens drive up expenditures, while the continuing absence of coverage for much of the population drives down the quality of the outcomes.

Table 1.4: Sources of spending on healthcare, 2020 (in percentage)

Out of Pocket	9.4
Private Health Insurance	27.9
Public Health Insurance[1]	40.2
Other[2]	22.5

[1] Including Medicare, Medicaid, CHIP (the Children's Health Insurance Program), Department of Veterans Affairs and Department of Defense.

[2] Includes Indian Health Services, research expenditures, public health programs and other state and local programs.

Yet a third paradox in American healthcare is that a system that is discussed as being private is actually more than half funded by the public sector. Public funding includes insurance such as Medicare and Medicaid, direct provision of services for veterans and native Americans, and through state and local governments, public health services at all three levels of government, health research, and a host of other programs. The health insurance purchased through the Affordable Care Act is subsidized although provided by private insurers,[2] but it has increased substantially the impact of the public sector on American healthcare.

Table 1.4 shows the distribution of spending for healthcare in the United States, and shows clearly the importance of the public sector. Just over a third of total health spending is now private, and this includes private health insurance bought through the Affordable Care Act that may be publicly subsidized. The large "other" category in this table is also heavily public, with a good deal of health research being paid for by the public sector, as well as public health and regulation programs (see Chapter 6) at all levels of government. The US system of healthcare is often referred to as being "private", but that is far from the reality.

This distribution of expenditures in Table 1.4 to some extent understates the impact of the public sector in spending. Some of the impact of government comes through the tax system rather than through expenditures per se. In particular, when an employer provides health insurance for his or her employees, they are in essence providing income, but that income is not taxed. In addition, provided they spend a sufficient amount relative to their income the amount individuals spend for healthcare can be deducted from income tax. In 2019 tax expenditures for healthcare were $234 billion, versus $1.2 trillion in direct expenditures. This hidden welfare state (Howard, 2006) is especially important for middle- and upper-income taxpayers who pay higher rates of tax.

Despite the impact of the public sector and its expenditures, the private sector still in many ways defines the manner in which the healthcare system functions. Although public, Medicare functions very much like a private insurance program, with deductibles and co-pays used as sources of finance, and as means of reducing consumption. Given that this program was designed for the elderly who have very large health expenditures on average and who also have fixed incomes, this was almost certainly a poor design (Davis and Schoen, 1978), but it reflects the power of the private sector ideas in thinking about health policy. Likewise, the insurance obtained through the Affordable Care Act is private, so that the insured also have out-of-pocket expenses when they use the program.

Following on from the third paradox, there is the apparent contradiction that a healthcare system with such a strong private sector flavor should be so much at the center of American political life. Many of the most important political battles over the past several decades have been over healthcare issues, including the numerous attempts to repeal the Affordable Care Act and the Supreme Court cases on its constitutionality. And the pandemic beginning in 2020 emphasized the role of the public sector in preparing for health emergencies and being capable of managing them when they occur. After the crisis of COVID-19 passes, there will be a need to reconsider the poor quality of the response, especially at the federal level, and the role of government in healthcare in the future. In particular, there is a need to strengthen public health capacity, and to restore public trust in institutions such as the Centers for Disease Control and Prevention that has been weakened by the pandemic (Commonwealth Fund, 2022a). And, finally, the battle over abortion rights, leading up to the Supreme Court decision of *Dobbs v Jackson Women's Health Organization*, has been a struggle over healthcare, as well as over the place of religion in American political life.

Healthcare and medical care

Although it may be discussed as healthcare, and this book is entitled health policy, it is important to remember that none of the medical providers mentioned above can really deliver health—they can deliver medical care but, in what Aaron Wildavsky (2018) called the "Great Equation", medicine does not equal health. Medicine can contribute to health, but it cannot guarantee health. Individual health also depends on other factors such as nutrition, exercise, housing and a host of other factors (Alderwick and Gottlieb, 2019). In the tables on infant mortality and life expectancy, the good performance of some countries such as Japan may be a function of lifestyle factors as much as the technical quality of the healthcare industry

Wildavsky's equation is a relatively moderate statement compared to some other analysis of contemporary "healthcare". The most extreme has come from Ivan Illich (1975) who argues that modern medicine does not contribute to health in a significant way, or at least not to the extent that is often assumed. In this view, modern medicine has reduced or eliminated the self-reliance of individuals, and made them dependent on medicine for their health. He further argues that modern medicine is iatrogenic, that is, harm producing.

Llich's emphasis on the harm of modern medicine is as much about the harm to society as it is to individuals. The harm to individuals is primarily that they lose their self-reliance and come to depend on the medical establishment to manage their health rather than making their own choices. The individual may believe that they do anything they wish—overeat, not exercise, drink alcohol to excess, smoke—without worry because modern medicine will take care of the problem. This is, of course, an overstatement on Illich's part, but it does emphasize the difference between medicine and health.

Illich's arguments may appear extreme to many practitioners of the medical professions and to most ordinary patients. He was clearly writing with an ideological perspective, but there are important points about how we approach health policy that should be considered. More recently, Barbara Ehrenreich (2018) has argued that the contemporary emphasis on "wellness" in society has pushed individuals to invest excessively in healthcare and medications of all types. Ehrenreich argues that individuals make those investments in the obviously misguided hope that they can avoid death, and the problems of aging. Ehrenreich echoes the adage that Americans believe death is negotiable.

Both Illich and Ehrenreich confirm Wildavsky's basic point about the disjuncture between health and medicine, albeit in a more dramatic fashion. But these analyses also point to another of Wildavsky's (2018) arguments about medicine and healthcare—that the demand for these services is essentially insatiable. His argument is that individuals want to live as long as they can, be as healthy as they can be during their lives, and perhaps have some plastic surgery to become more physically attractive. If there are no financial, or other, constraints, then individuals will tend to consume large quantities of medical care. The question is whether consumption of medical care will actually lead to better health?

Even if the patient is not pursuing their own health and longevity, the medical system itself may produce something of the same outcomes of high levels of consumption of medical care. Wildavsky's "Medical Uncertainty Principle" asserts that there is always one more test that can be made to attempt to eliminate some of the uncertainty for the patient, and perhaps especially the doctor.[3] Some doctors are beginning to recognize that routine testing often leads to more testing, with no clear evidence of improving the quality of life of the patient. Likewise, unnecessary surgery is an endemic problem in American healthcare (Outcalt, 2021), However, as long as money is available then spending, the testing, and the procedures will continue. While value-based medicine (Burwell, 2015), and the power of insurance companies, is placing some constraints on procedures and the level of spending, there are still pressures for more service, and for more spending.

The demand from patients for a healthier and longer life, combined with pressures from the healthcare industry itself, tends to produce increased spending and consumption. Some of the demand for medical care is also created by advertising from pharmaceutical companies, and from healthcare providers such as hospitals, who promote the newest and (presumably) most effective treatments for a variety of diseases. As I will point out below, the pressures from advertising can lead to the replacement of perfectly adequate existing medications with newer and more expensive ones, with little gain for the patient.

All three of the authors discussed in this section, albeit Wildavsky to a lesser extent, are arguing that individual patients are to some extent being misled by the healthcare, or "wellness", industry into spending too much of their money and time in medical care. Now that hospitals and drug companies can advertise their products and services, medical care has become to an extent like other products, and demand is being created. Of course, these advertisements may have been pushing at an open door, as individuals want to be as healthy as possible, and the advertising may simply give them ideas about how and where they can achieve the higher level of health being sought.

While one cannot, and should not, deny the importance of advances of modern medicine, these three authors also remind us that much of the progress in longevity and health quality for individuals is the product of public health measures and prevention, rather than curative medicine. What we now consider in developed countries as normal facts of life—clean water and sanitation—have saved many more lives than even "wonder drugs" such as penicillin.[4] Vaccinations have now eliminated diseases that once killed and afflicted millions.

The importance of public health and very basic aspects of healthcare have been highlighted by the COVID-19 crisis. One of the major weapons against the virus has been one of the oldest—washing hands regularly. And an old tool of coping with contagious diseases such as tuberculosis and syphilis (Barry, 2020)—contact tracing—has been shown to be effective in controlling the spread of the virus. The public health system in the United States had been degraded by lowered expenditures over the past decade at least, and the capacity to respond with contact tracing and public health interventions was relatively poor (Watson et al., 2017).

The COVID-19 pandemic provided additional evidence about the impacts, or perhaps lack thereof, of modern medicine. In a survey performed concerning the period of May to July, 2020, 41 percent of respondents in the United States reported they had put off planned medical appointments or interventions because of the virus or because their usual provider was closed (Henry, 2021). Despite that, the vast majority reported no difference in their health, and some reported that their health was actually better (see Lawrence, 2020). Perhaps especially interesting was that the group who saw the least negative effects on health during the crisis were senior citizens, who are usually major consumers of healthcare. The above said, however, people with serious conditions who avoided treatments did apparently die in large numbers (Thebault et al., 2020).

Three images of American healthcare

I will present three alternative models of American healthcare in an attempt to understand the nature of the contemporary practice of medicine and healthcare, and the public policies that help to maintain it. Whenever one attempts to encapsulate an entity as large and diffuse as American healthcare in a simple image there is an obvious chance, if not certainty, of oversimplifying. Still, beginning with these images in mind is a means of putting large amounts of information into manageable categories.

The jungle

The first image of American healthcare is that it is a jungle. Health policy in the United States, and indeed every other country, is complex and is difficult to understand. Some of the complexity is a function of the nature of healthcare itself, involving a good deal of advanced science. In the United States the technical nature and complexity of the production of healthcare is exacerbated by the large number of actors involved in delivering the services, and their numerous interactions. It is easy to become lost in all that complexity, just as an adventurer may become lost in a real jungle.

The major group of actors lost in the jungle are the patients. They come to the healthcare system seeking treatment for their illnesses or perhaps just a simple checkup to be sure that they are indeed healthy. To say they come to a system implies, however, more organization than many patients say they find as they seek medical care. In one recent survey (PHRMA, 2022) 40 percent of the respondents said they did not know what was covered by their insurance, and almost 80 percent said there were too many barriers to getting their needed medications.[5] The patients must confront numerous rules, that sometimes conflict, about payment for the providers, the availability of drugs and procedures, and numerous other components of their care. They also have to sort through recommendations for treatment and decide what is best for them—generally without any medical training.

But patients are not the only ones lost in this jungle. Although often seen as the most powerful creatures in the jungle, doctors are increasingly having to fight their way through the jungle to be able to perform their jobs and to serve their patients. The jungle that doctors confront is largely the creation of the insurance industry. It involves numerous reimbursement rules and forms that differ among the insurers, as well as different formularies for the drugs that can be prescribed. Further, given that an increasing number of doctors are employed by hospitals which have their own rules, the jungle may be becoming more dense and impenetrable. Doctors and their employees report having to spend hours each week fighting their way through those rules, while attempting to provide the best possible care to the patients.

Doctors also encounter difficulties in coordinating among themselves and in providing integrated care to their patients. A study by the Commonwealth Fund (see Doty et al., 2020) found that primary care physicians in the United States struggled more than some other consolidated democracies to coordinate care for their patients with specialists (see Table 1.5). This is true even though most physicians are now employed in networks that presumably provide more integrated care. Likewise, US doctors were much less likely to link their patients with social services than were doctors in other countries. Both the doctor and the patient therefore are acting independently rather than as part of a more integrated system of care.

In short, for many people involved in healthcare the process of seeking care, or delivering care, has become extremely convoluted and confusing. The simple process of a patient seeing his or her doctor and that doctor having the clinical

Table 1.5: Percentage of primary physicians who receive information from specialists about changes to patients' care plans or medications

Germany	27
Sweden	42
Netherlands	43
US	49
Australia	57
Canada	58
Switzerland	60
UK	69
Norway	70
France	73
New Zealand	77

Source: Doty et al. (2020).

freedom to make a diagnosis and then prescribe a treatment is now encumbered by numerous rules and procedures that appear to hinder rather than facilitate delivering care to the patient. This jungle nature of contemporary healthcare is not just an inconvenience. It may prevent patients from receiving the care they need in a timely manner, and it is a leading cause of doctors leaving the practice of medicine.

The jungle metaphor may apply to more than just the difficulties confronted by individual patients when confronting the healthcare system The public sector in the United States is complex and all levels of government are involved in healthcare in one way or another. And even at the federal level there are multiple organizations that have some role in providing or regulating healthcare (see Table 1.6). Thus, attempting to determine what health policy is may involve putting together a number of different positions and programs and trying to find the coherence among them.

The intergovernmental jungle in healthcare has been demonstrated all too clearly in coping with the COVID-19 crisis in 2020. Although there was an expectation that the federal government would have the primary responsibility for managing the crisis, in practice state and local governments played a significant, if not dominant, role in providing healthcare and in developing plans for containing the outbreak (Gordon et al., 2020). The policy and administrative issues in managing the crisis were complicated by political differences among the governments (Blake, 2020), and governors and mayors reported themselves entangled in complicated intergovernmental policy disputes over policy and the availability of resources.

As well as reflecting the federalism of American government, the jungle model of healthcare also reflects the difficulties in making policy given the separation of powers within the federal government, and the general incremental

Table 1.6: Government organizations active in healthcare

Federal		
	Health and Human Services	Medicare, Medicaid, CHIPs, FDA
	Defense	Military and Military Dependents Healthcare
	Veterans Affairs	VA Hospitals
	Interior	Native Americans Health Service
	Labor	Occupational Safety and Health
	Homeland Security	Bioterrorism
	Agriculture	Food Inspection
	State	WHO, PAHO
State (Pennsylvania)		
	State Health Department	Regulating Nursing Homes
		Health Promotion
		Community Health
	Department of Human Services	State Hospitals
	Department of Agriculture	Food Inspection
Local (Allegheny County)		
	County Health Department	Immunizations
		Public Health
		Restaurant Inspection

Note: CHIPs = Children's Health Insurance Program; FDA = Food and Drug Administration; PAHO = Pan-American Health Organization; VA = Veterans Affairs; WHO = World Health Organization.

style of policymaking in the United States. The constitutional separation of powers, especially given the strong partisan divisions at present, makes passing comprehensive legislation difficult. Further, when they do occur—as in the case of the Affordable Care Act—major policy innovations tend to involve multiple concessions to multiple interests that make the subsequent implementation of the law more difficult—for the bureaucracy and for citizens.

A hierarchy

The second image in healthcare in the United States is that of a hierarchy. The hierarchy may be no better for the patients than the jungle. In the hierarchical conception of healthcare, rather than being a chaotic interaction of actors, there is a single actor that is a "hierarch" and can exercise control over the entire healthcare system. The question then becomes which among at least three possible candidates for that central position is actually in control. In some ways, that may make little difference to the patients who are subject to the control with little power of their own.

The first candidate for the hierarch is the medical profession. For most of the history of healthcare in the United States doctors would have been in charge and were clearly the hierarch. They could exercise clinical freedom and tended to have a god-like status with their patients and the other groups of actors involved in the healthcare industry. Despite the historical power of the medical profession in healthcare, that power now seems diminished substantially, with it being transferred to the two other possible hierarchs.

That said, the claims for clinical freedom remain important. The medical profession ultimately makes most decisions about patient care, and attempts to alter that control over the practice of medicine are resisted vigorously by medical organizations, and by patients if they are aware that an insurance company is interfering with their treatment. As important as clinical freedom may be for the practice of medicine, there is some evidence that it can lead to slowed innovation, and inadequate use of information in decisions about treatments (Patashnik et al., 2017).

The second possible hierarch in healthcare are the health insurance companies. As the financing of healthcare has become a more crucial element in the American system, insurance companies have been able to gain power over the rest of the system. Sixty-six percent of the American population has private health insurance; private insurance payments are higher than those of public health insurance— Medicare and Medicaid—and hence their policyholders are more important to doctors and to hospitals. The insurance companies are powerful not only because of the reimbursements per se but also because they influence other aspects of medical practice.

The third candidate for the hierarchical controller of the healthcare system is government. Like the private insurers, government is a major funder of healthcare, both through insurance for individuals, direct funding for healthcare for groups such as veterans and native Americans, and through funding medical research. In addition, government is a major regulator of the healthcare industry, including the pharmaceutical industry, hospitals and many aspects of individual access to healthcare provision. The role of government has been important for decades but has been increased through legislation, such as the Health Insurance Portability and Accountability Act 1996 (HIPAA) and especially the Affordable Care Act.

The choice of which of these three candidates is the hierarch and, indeed, whether the system is a hierarchy at all, is very much in the eye of beholder. There are some arguments to be made for each of the three candidates. Each may be a hierarch in some aspects of healthcare. Doctors, for example, may be in charge when actually treating patients, until, of course, they confront insurance companies that attempt to control the drugs they prescribe, or the procedures they implement. The insurance companies may appear to be in charge in many situations, but may be regulated by government and must depend on doctors and hospitals to deliver the services their policy holders have contracted for. And government can regulate and can fund, but also depends on others in the system to deliver the products and services.

America has the best healthcare in the world

The third image of healthcare in the United States is that it is the best healthcare system in the world. This positive image may be difficult to sustain, given some of the evidence presented earlier in this chapter, but it is widely proclaimed by Americans and especially by American politicians. The proponents of this view point to the modern hospitals, the amount of medical research, and the quality of American medical education as evidence for the success of the healthcare system.

There is some firmer evidence to support the contention that American healthcare is the best of the world. One of the strongest pieces of evidence is the survival rates for several cancers in the United States compared to other industrial democracies. Table 1.7 shows that, for all the types of cancer, listed survival rates in the United States are higher than in most other countries of the world, including Canada and the major European countries. In some instances, the differences are not large, but the United States does perform well on this measure of performance that may be more directly related to the healthcare system than infant mortality or life expectancy.

The poor infant mortality figures for the United States have been a major indictment of the system, but if looked at different they can be considered much

Table 1.7: Cancer survival rates, 2022

	Type of Cancer		
	Breast	Stomach	Lung
United States	88.6	29.1	18.7
Brazil	87.4	24.9	18.0
France	86.9	27.7	13.6
Finland	86.6	25.2	12.3
Australia	86.2	27.9	15.0
Sweden	86.2	23.2	15.6
Canada	85.8	24.8	17.3
Germany	85.3	31.6	16.2
Japan	84.7	54.0	30.0
Denmark	82.0	17.9	11.3
United Kingdom	81.1	18.5	9.6
Poland	74.1	18.6	13.4
India	60.4	18.7	9.6

Source: CONCORD Programme, London School of Hygiene and Tropical Medicine.

Table 1.8: Index of health science and technology, 2020

United States	75.1
Denmark	52.6
Netherlands	50.0
Sweden	49.7
United Kingdom	49.4
Singapore	48.0
Switzerland	47.3
Germany	46.9
Finland	46.8
Belgium	44.9

Source: *FREOPP World Index of Healthcare Innovation,* https://freopp.org/united-states-health-system-prof ile-4-in-the-world-index-of-healthcare-innovation-b593ba15a96.

more positively. The infant mortality rates in Table 1.2 are totals for all live births. If, however, we look at the details of those infant deaths, the picture of American healthcare is more positive. First, the United States uses a definition of live births that counts some premature births that would be excluded in many statistical systems. Further, the survival of premature babies is better in the United States than in many countries.

Although not measuring the actual delivery of health services, there are several other indicators that could support an argument that US healthcare is the best in the world. One is the amount of medical research that is conducted in the United States. Although many other countries are also heavily engaged in research, the United States invests substantially in medical research. Much of this research is funded by government, especially the federal government, but a good deal of research is also funded by the private sector, for example the pharmaceutical industry. The rate of innovation in medical science in the United States has been extremely high, and that has translated into extremely high levels of capability within the system. The United States rates as number one on an international index of scientific innovation in healthcare (Table 1.8), but the score for healthcare is lowered overall because of problems of access and fiscal sustainability (Girvan and Roy, 2020).

Another important indicator of quality, especially for patients, is waiting time (Table 1.9). How long does a patient have to wait before seeing his or her physician, or seeing a specialist? How long does it take for the patient to hear back from the doctor about a question or a test? While waiting times may not necessarily determine the final outcome of the encounter with the medical system, long waiting times do give the impression of low quality service, and may impose more pain and anxiety on the patient. Waiting times for seeing specialists in the United States are among the best in the developed countries, but waiting times for hearing back from the doctor are much less positive.

Table 1.9: Waiting times, 2022

	Waiting time to see specialist (% more than one month)	Waiting time to hear back from doctor (% less than one day)
Switzerland	23	12
Germany	25	13
Netherlands	25	13
United States	27	28
Australia	39	14
United Kingdom	41	21
New Zealand	48	17
Sweden	52	24
Canada	61	33

Source: OECD, *Waiting Times for Healthcare Services*, https://www.oecd.org/els/health-systems/waiting-times.htm.

Even with the positive evidence we can identify for the quality of healthcare in the United States, the experience of the COVID-19 pandemic revealed a number of deficiencies in the system. On the one hand, the treatment of patients once diagnosed and being treated was generally very good, at least in the major medical centers. On the other hand, factors within the health system led to a very large number of cases, and major shortages of personal protective equipment, virus tests and ventilators to treat the most severe cases. Further, the regional and racial disparities in contracting the disease, and in outcomes for those infected by the virus, were marked (Alcendor, 2020).

Perhaps the conclusion that can be drawn from these various pieces of information about the quality of healthcare in the United States is that there is extremely high quality medical care available but it is not available to everyone. Even after the adoption of the Affordable Care Act millions of Americans are not covered by health insurance, and millions more lack adequate coverage. Many people have health insurance that has high deductibles and co-payments, making it expensive to use. And there may well be other barriers, such as regional disparities, that prevent effective consumption of medical services.

Politics of health policy

Much of the politics of health policy in the United States can be seen as conflicts between those three images of healthcare, and especially conflicts between and within the first two—the jungle and hierarchy. Some actors want to maintain a disaggregated, assumedly competitive, arrangement for healthcare, because their interests can thrive in that setting. But the hierarchical actors want to rationalize the healthcare system and create a better organized system by imposing their values and priorities on the system.

The principal actors wanting to maintain the jungle may be the medical professions. While Robert Alford (1975) referred to doctors, nurses and other medical practitioners as "professional monopolists", they actually do well in a more decentralized, fragmented system because they can have a great deal of individual power over patients, and over other actors such as hospitals. This pattern of professional dominance prevailed until the insurance companies began to gain control over many aspects of healthcare, including some aspects of the clinical freedom of physicians, for example influencing which medications will be prescribed.

There are also conflicts among the potential hierarchs within healthcare. While physicians might have been the hierarchs at some point in time, they have lost that position to either the health insurance companies and/or government. In contemporary healthcare politics there has been an ongoing conflict between government and the insurers, with the passage of Obamacare being one major victory for government. "Big Pharma", the pharmaceutical industry, also plays the role of hierarch in some important parts of the system, with government also attempting to assert control over pricing of drugs.

Hospitals were once major contenders for the hierarch in the system, but they have lost a good deal of their influence for several reasons. The first, and most important, is the power of the insurance industry in setting reimbursement rates, coupled with the power of government to set rates through Medicare and Medicaid. Further, the growth of independent surgical centers and other ambulatory care opportunities has moved a good deal of income-producing activity away from hospitals. That said, hospitals have been able to make something of a comeback in their relative power by hiring physicians directly, gaining more control over them, and over the revenues they produce.

These structural conflicts among powerful actors in healthcare are likely to continue, especially with government possibly continuing to attempt to exert more control. Popular support for a larger role for government in health, even after the adoption of the Affordable Care Act (see Chapter 5), will drive some of that conflict. There will also be pressures for government to confront the power of the pharmaceutical industry and do something about the high and increasing prices of prescription drugs. In all these policy battles the public—in their roles as citizens and consumers—are perhaps the least powerful actors (see Giaimo, 2009) .

Federalism represents another important structural factor in American healthcare policy. Historically, health policy has been dominated by state governments, with the federal government becoming a significant player only in the 1950s. Even then the states were responsible for most aspects of health, especially any provision of services to the public through facilities such as public hospitals and visiting nurses. The states continue to play a major role in health policy, and were major actors during the pandemic, especially early when the Trump administration essentially turned the crisis over to the states (Peters, 2022). This period also pointed out the possibilities of conflict in health policy, and other policies, when different political parties control the federal government and state governments.

The fragmentation in public policies resulting from federalism is exacerbated by fragmentation within the institutions of government. The separation of powers inherent in the US Constitution makes decision-making ponderous, and often impossible. The passage of the Affordable Care Act during a rare period of unified government (both houses of Congress and the presidency controlled by the same party), and the health provisions of the Inflation Reduction Act, represent rare instances of the ability to push through major legislation (but see Polsby, 1985). Any major reform of health policy will involve opportunities for building coalitions across parties and party factions that rarely occur.

In addition to the structural conflicts among actors involved in health policy, there has been increasing partisan politics that has extended beyond the fight over the Affordable Care Act. This conflict was very apparent during the pandemic, with many Republican politicians rejecting the scientific advice from major institutions in favor of home remedies, or even total denial of the pandemic's danger to the public. It has also extended to the use of fetal cells in medical research, given the alleged connection between abortion and fetal cells.[6] These partisan conflicts run the risk of undermining the quality of medical care provided, and the research needed for new cures.

Partisan politics is accompanied by a great deal of involvement of interest groups in healthcare policy. All the major actors in this policy area are represented by well-funded and active interest groups that represent their members in Washington and in the state capitols (see Table 1.10; see also Callahan, 2009). There are also numerous interest groups advocating for more research into various diseases, many of which also fund research on their own. The group least well represented in the complex world of health policy are ordinary patients. The major advocacy group for patients has been the American Association of Retired Persons (AARP) that has a particular interest in Medicare. That said, AARP has the largest membership of any interest group in the United States (38 million).

The central trichotomy: access, cost and quality

The politics of healthcare in the United States, and arguably in any political system, involves coping with three variables that define the nature of the system. These three variables are access, cost and quality. The first concern for many policymakers is ensuring access—ensuring the people who need medical care can get it. In all other consolidated democracies, access is largely ensured through public sector programs that either provide the medical care directly or that provide insurance so citizens can get the medical care they require (see Chapter 2). That level of access does not exist in the United States, and millions of people lack proper health insurance.

The second variable is cost. How much does it cost—both government and private actors—to provide healthcare? If Wildavsky and other analysts are correct that the demand for healthcare is virtually insatiable then cost is going to be a persistent problem in all healthcare systems. Many spend less than does the United

Table 1.10: Examples of interest groups in health policy in the United States

Professional
American Medical Association
American Nursing Association
American Medical Technologists
Other Providers
American Hospital Association
Ambulatory Surgery Care Association
Health Insurance
Blue Cross-Blue Shield Association
American Health Insurance Plans
Pharmaceuticals (Mostly Individual Companies)
Pfizer
AMGEN
Patients
American Association of Retired Persons
Other
Biotechnology Innovation Organization

States, but that is still a major object of spending. Further, demand is not the only factor affecting cost, as the supply of technological innovations (including new pharmaceuticals) has a major influence on costs (Callahan, 2009), as do a number of other factors (see Chapter 8). Cost is especially important in the United States given the extremely high level of spending on healthcare.

The third of these major variables for healthcare is quality. Access is important, but if the quality of the healthcare being delivered to patients is not good then the positive effects of access may be reduced. Assessing the quality of healthcare is difficult, despite the common use of indicators such as infant mortality and cancer survival rates. Further, to some extent the quality of healthcare is in the eye of the beholder—the patient. Even if healthcare is technically correct the patient may not like it if delivered in an impersonal and seemingly uncaring manner.

The difficulty for anyone attempting to manage a healthcare system is that these three variables tend to be trade-offs. If access is emphasized, and more patients are treated, then costs will increase and quality may be affected by overcrowding. Likewise, if cost control is emphasized by decision-makers then access is likely to be reduced and quality also negatively affected. And if quality is the primary value then fewer people may be treated (although perhaps treated better) and costs will increase. As I discuss various major programs in US healthcare policy, and the details of these three major variables, the need to make trade-offs will be a theme that will appear a number of times.

Conclusion

The various images that exist of American healthcare are contradictory and paradoxical. The high-tech image of glistening urban hospitals can be contrasted with the rather dingy nature of facilities in poor and rural areas—assuming they exist at all. The public sector has assumed responsibility for healthcare for the majority of Americans now, but the model through which it is delivered, and the service providers, are largely private. The one aspect of the system that appears clear is that healthcare in the United States is extremely expensive, and is increasingly expensive.

The remainder of this book will attempt to make sense of the complexities of health policy in the United States. The focus will be on the policies themselves, but these policies will be discussed within the context of the politics that shape them. I will first compare US health policies with other countries, with an emphasis on the greater ease of access for citizens in other democratic systems. I will then proceed to discuss four major policies—Medicare, Medicaid, the Affordable Care Act and a collection of regulatory programs—that comprise the major interventions of the federal government into healthcare. I will then discuss each of the three major variables—access, cost and quality—mentioned above in greater detail, and will end with a discussion of possible developments in this policy area—especially the possibility of truly universal coverage.

The question of universal health insurance raises perhaps the fundamental question about health policy in the United States. Is healthcare a basic right of citizenship, or is it a commodity that is purchased in the market, or is it a privilege that some members of society receive from government and others do not? Existing policies provide a "yes" answer to all of these questions, although the answer for a right applies only to a limited range of medical services such as emergency rooms. The debate over single-payer plans in the 2020 presidential election put the question of rights more clearly in the political spotlight, but definitive acceptance of that right still appears improbable in the near future.

2

American healthcare in comparative perspective

American healthcare policy is substantially different from healthcare in other consolidated democracies. The discussion in the previous chapter characterized the American system in analytic terms, and this chapter will provide more description. Further, that description will be compared with six other wealthy countries that provide their citizens healthcare in different ways. I will also discuss some elements of government and society in the United States that help to explain why the greater reliance on private sector provision of healthcare persists. Some of the points about the US system developed in this chapter will be developed in greater detail in the remaining chapters of this book.

American healthcare system

I will now discuss five important features of the US health system that help to explain some of the outcomes of the system. These characteristics also provide a basis for comparing the other healthcare systems with that of the United States, and they also help to demonstrate the need for continuing reforms of health policy in the United States. The structural features of the healthcare system are such that even the skills and good intentions of individuals working within the system are incapable of preventing the less positive outcomes in infant mortality and life expectancy discussed in Chapter 1.

A mixed system of finance and delivery

The factor that distinguishes healthcare in the United States from other similar countries is the role played by the private sector in financing and delivery of healthcare. Although I have shown (Table 1.4) that financing of healthcare is now more than half public, there is still a significant amount of private financing. That private financing is in the form of insurance, as well as in the out-of-pocket expenses paid by the insured in both public and private health insurance programs. Likewise, although almost half of Americans are insured through some public sector program such as Medicare or Medicaid, millions are also insured privately. Most citizens who receive their insurance from their employer as a benefit of employment tend to be attached to that insurance, and tend to be hesitant about further public involvement in health insurance (Hamel et al., 2019). Many of the privately insured support something like "Medicare for All", provided they can keep their own insurance (see Chapter 10). As employers move toward high deductible plans because of the costs of better plans, that level of satisfaction of employees with private insurance is declining. Even many of those counted here as having private insurance are receiving subsidies through the Affordable Care Act, pointing out that the mixture between public and private is pervasive.

When I say "private" in the above paragraph, that term includes both for-profit and not-for-profit providers. Much of private health insurance is written by for-profit providers, including very large firms such as the Hartford, Cigna and Aetna. In 2020 these private insurers made a collective profit of $36 billion, much of it now coming from Medicare Part C (see Chapter 3). There are some not-for-profit insurers, notably Blue Cross-Blue Shield programs that were originally organized by the medical profession to insure their patients. There are, however, debates and law suits over exactly how non-profit these insurers are, as they have billions of dollars of "retained earnings" each year. In many cases the behavior of the for-profit and the not-for-profit providers are indistinguishable.

The providers of healthcare services are also a mixture of public, for-profit, and not-for-profit actors. The proportion of public providers is much smaller than the proportion of public sector expenditure, but there are public hospitals, public clinics and public health professionals delivering services. The largest examples of public service providers are the Departments of Veterans Affairs and the Department of Defense facilities, and the services providing healthcare to native Americans. Not-for-profits are major providers of health services, including many hospitals (almost half of the total) as well as clinics in disadvantaged areas. Finally, there are hospitals and other facilities that operate for profit, with one-quarter of hospitals being for profit.

Despite this mixture of providers and the majority public funding, much of the ethos of the healthcare system remains largely private. The Affordable Care Act uses for-profit insurers for much of its insurance. Medicare Parts C and D are provided by private insurers, and insurance through the Affordable Care Act uses co-payments and deductibles both to help finance the services and to deter consumption. Not-for-profit providers often appear to operate in the same way as do for-profit providers, with high salaries for executives and fees that tend to be close to or equal to for-profit providers. The healthcare system is formally mixed public–private, but tends to think in terms of dollars and cents as much as in terms of providing a public service.

A fragmented and decentralized system

The financing and delivery of healthcare is fragmented between the public and the private sectors, and it is further fragmented by levels of government. American federalism influences the provision of programs, even federally-funded programs, and this in turn means that the system is more decentralized than are healthcare systems in many other countries. That fragmentation and decentralization results in different levels of access for citizens depending upon their state of residence. It further increases costs of managing healthcare, just as the differences among types of providers also increases costs.

Medicare is the only truly national health insurance program. The availability of traditional Medicare is the same no matter where the person lives. Even for Medicare, however, there are differences in the availability of Part C programs (Medicare Advantage) and Part D (Prescription Drugs) in different states, or even in different parts of the same state. Also, "Medigap insurance", which fills in for the deficiencies in Medicare coverage, differs across states.[1] Further, some states subsidize low-income Medicare recipients more than do others. This high level of decentralization means that citizens may be disadvantaged by their residence and, further, that they have to do a good deal of shopping if they want to take advantage of programs.

Fee-for-service medicine

Paying for medical care on a fee-for-service basis is one of the key features of American medical care. In most cases each service provided to a patient is billed separately, and the income of most physicians varies depending upon the number of patients they see, and the number of procedures they perform. Revenues for hospitals and other providers are also determined by services rendered. Fee-for-service medicine is often seen as one of the causes of the high level of spending for healthcare in the United States, given that providers always have a financial incentive to do more.

Several mechanisms have been used to attempt to overcome problems in fee-for-service provision. The most common is managed care, in which primary care physicians (PCPs) function as gatekeepers and patients must be referred to specialists and other services through the PCP. In managed care programs there are generally networks of physicians and hospitals who have agreed to a schedule of fees from each insurer, and patients will have to pay much more if they want to go to an out-of-network provider. Over time, some of the constraints on patients in managed care have been loosened because of their unpopularity with patients (see Orentlicher, 2003).

Health Maintenance Organizations (HMOs) are the other major alternative to conventional fee-for-service medicine. In this system the patient pays an annual fee for all his or her medical care. The HMO is then responsible for providing that care without additional fees. This system also restricts the providers the patient can use, and gives those providers an incentive *not* to treat, or *not* to do tests, so as not to exhaust the fees that have already been paid. That incentive is good for cost containment (see Chapter 8), but may not be good for the health of the patient.

Fee-for-service medicine is practiced in most of the healthcare systems that are discussed in the remainder of this chapter, albeit without the extremely high rates of growth of spending on healthcare. The major difference is that there are caps on the amount of money which a provider can earn in a month or a year, and/or monitoring of the levels of billing by individual providers. Fee-for-service medicine does set the tone for healthcare in the United States, but the effects of this payment system on expenditures could be controlled with more government intervention.[2]

A regulated system, with many holes

The discussion of insurance and the provision of health services above covers many crucial programs in American health policy, but also leaves out important regulatory programs. All levels of government are involved in regulating some aspects of providing services. The federal government, for example, regulates the licensing of pharmaceuticals, as well as many other aspects of healthcare after legislation such as the Affordable Care Act and the Health Insurance Portability and Accountability Act (HIPAA) have been adopted. State governments license facilities such as hospitals and nursing homes,[3] and also are responsible for professional licensing. Local governments may also license facilities, as well as attempting to control diseases by inspecting restaurants, grocery stores, etc. Local governments also provide public health services such as vaccinations and monitoring of specified diseases.

While public regulation is, like the rest of the system, rather fragmented, there is also a good deal of private regulation or self-regulation in the system. Although the states license doctors, nurses and other professionals to practice, much of the certification of their qualifications is done privately through medical associations. The states also regulate health insurance, and after *Dobbs v Jackson Women's Health Organization* many will regulate abortion in a very severe manner. Likewise, hospital and nursing home accreditation is done privately and the private inspection functions in parallel with state licensing. This fragmentation of regulation is another source of cost within the system, given the administrative burdens involved.

Despite the number of regulators involved already, there may also be holes in the regulations. The Food and Drug Administration does not have as close supervision of drugs after they are licensed as some critics deem desirable. Further, they have very limited control over dietary supplements that are marketed as improving health and addressing some specific health problems. Finally, there are a number of aspects of charging patients and their insurers that are not well-regulated, especially the billing for services out of networks controlled by an insurance company. Some of the most egregious forms of "surprise billing" are now regulated, but patients continue to find themselves with huge bills for services they believed were covered by insurance (Keith et al., 2022).

An unequal system

Finally, in part because of some of the features already mentioned, the American healthcare system contains a large number of inequalities for individuals. In the chapters that follow I will detail differential levels of access, and differential outcomes, that occur based on race, ethnicity and gender. These differences have become more politically visible during the past several years, and there are now more efforts in place to attempt to reduce the disparities that occur. The programs that have been introduced by governments, professional organizations, individual hospitals and other actors are having to change patterns of unequal treatment that have been in place for decades (Dickman et al., 2017).

There are also a number of inequalities in healthcare that are less visible politically, but no less important. For example, there are massive differences in access to healthcare, and in the quality of healthcare, between rural and urban areas. If anything, these differences have been becoming worse as rural areas continue to lose population and economic activity. Differences by area are also found among the states, with large differences between states in the Northeast and those in the South on variables such as infant mortality and life expectancy (WalletHub, 2022). Also, despite the obvious increase in the elderly population, the healthcare system has not been developing the resources needed for coping with aging patients, nor sufficient knowledge of the differences in how diseases and treatments affect elderly patients differently from younger patients.

The degree of inequality within the healthcare system of the United States can be seen by using the same indicator of infant mortality used to compare the United States to other countries. The infant mortality rate for African-Americans in 2019 was 10.5 deaths per 1,000 live births, while that for white Americans was 4.5. The infant mortality rate in Mississippi was 8.3, while that in California was 3.7.[4] The infant mortality rate for Black babies in Oklahoma was 13.4, slightly higher than that of Brazil. It is clear that the high-quality medicine available in the United States is not reaching all of its citizens.

Comparable healthcare systems

The rather negative description of the healthcare system of the United States can serve as the basis for describing other systems of paying for and delivering health services in other wealthy and democratic systems (see also Capano et al., 2022, ch. 4). Each of these systems would be worthy of a book-length treatment of its own, but that is not possible here; so I will only provide a sketch of these systems and what features distinguish them from that of the United States. The cases selected illustrate the major options used in providing healthcare, and in most cases there are other countries that are similarly organized.

United Kingdom

The healthcare system of the United Kingdom is the least like that of any of the wealthy countries, especially the United States. First, the National Health Service (NHS) is primarily public, albeit with a limited amount of private involvement. It is also centralized, with most decision-making and, more importantly, budget allocations, made in the center of government. The system is, however, implemented separately in Wales and Scotland through the Welsh and Scottish devolved governments (see, for example, Greer, 2016; Nottingham, 2019). In Northern Ireland, the healthcare system was created separately, but now is administered in much the same way as in the other three parts of the United Kingdom.

The NHS began functioning in 1948 to provide health services "free at the point of delivery". The NHS involves direct provision of health services, rather than being a primarily insurance-based system like the others we will discuss in this chapter. The NHS hires personnel, runs hospitals, and provides many other healthcare services. Although all citizens and legal residents in the United Kingdom are eligible for services through the NHS, some four million people also have private insurance—some provided by their employers as in the United States—and there are also "self-pay" patients who opt to pay for private services out of pocket. The opportunity for faster service and more up-market facilities attracts many citizens who can afford to utilize private sector health facilities.

The NHS in England is now organized into clinical commissioning groups responsible for specific areas of the country. Those groups are responsible for estimating what health services will be needed within that territory and then developing the capacity to meet those needs, within their budget. The budget constraints on the NHS are more genuine than those in US healthcare, and may pose significant challenges to managers. The budget for the NHS is a continuing issue in British politics, as is the capacity of the system to meet the needs of the public (see Ham, 2020). The problem of emergency services and waiting lists has been especially important as the pent-up demand from the time of the pandemic hits the NHS (Neville, 2023).

General practitioners (GPs) are primarily contract employees, although in some more remote parts of the United Kingdom, for example the Scottish islands, they may be public employees. GPs are paid on a capitation basis, and function as gatekeepers within the system. Although patients can self-refer to private specialists, they must get a referral from their GP for NHS consultants. Many NHS consultants also have private patients, although the amount they can earn in the private sector is limited. Other NHS staff—nurses, technicians, etc.—are direct employees of the organization.

Although basic medical services are free, other aspects of healthcare may not be totally free, depending upon where in the United Kingdom a person lives. In England, each prescription for individuals under 60 years of age costs £9.65 for a three months' supply. Prescription drugs are free in the other parts of the United Kingdom. Vision examinations are free for people over 60, but most people will have to pay for eyeglasses. Dental examinations are also provided through the NHS, although most dentists also have private practices. Some basic dental treatments are funded, but more extensive and cosmetic treatment will require a fee.

Although exemplary in providing access to healthcare for citizens, the NHS is not without its problems. One has been the continuing reform and reorganization of the service, attempting to find *the* solution to the problem of providing increasingly complex and expensive medical services to the population within a fixed budget. This has created "reform fatigue" among many participants in the system and, as Rudolf Klein (1999) argued, often does not allow a fair test of the reforms.

Waiting times are another continuing problem for the NHS. The official maximum waiting time to see a specialist is 18 weeks, but in the summer of 2022 the waiting time could be much longer. As of June 2022 there were 6.73 million people waiting for appointments, with 2.54 million having been waiting more than the expected 18 weeks (BMA, 2022). Politically, waiting times tend to be used as a gauge of the commitment of a government to the health service, and its management capacities.

Sweden

Swedish healthcare is also universal and delivered to citizens without an insurance program that charges premiums—taxes and co-pays fund the public system, which in turn provides most of the healthcare for the population. The Swedish system differs from the NHS in the United Kingdom by being much less centralized. The county (*län*) governments in Sweden are major players in healthcare, and local (*kommun*) governments are also involved, especially in the linkage between healthcare and social care. The entire system is overseen by the Health and Welfare Board (*Socialstyrelsen*) in the central government. This autonomous agency coordinates its activities with seven other agencies that are concerned with funding some parts of the overall healthcare system, as well as regulating the system (Strelenhert et al., 2015).

One of the important features of the system is the degree of political involvement in managing healthcare. The elected boards at the county and regional levels are responsible for making health policy for their regions, within the framework established nationally. This level of government is also responsible for collecting much of the revenue that is used to fund the healthcare system. The regions are especially important for managing and funding hospitals, with some implicit competition among them for the best healthcare. Likewise, the elected boards of municipalities can make their own policies about some aspects of healthcare, such as smaller clinics, nursing homes and home care, and fund these services. The central government does provide some grants for healthcare purposes, but finance as well as delivery is decentralized.

GPs are primarily contractors with government (through the regions) rather than direct employees, and are organized into approximately 1,100 delivery units around the country. Many are privately owned and operated, although some in more remote regions of the country will be publicly managed. These care centers are funded through three streams of income. First, they are paid on a capitation basis for patients registered with their practice, and they are also paid on a fee-for-service basis. Finally, they can earn small amounts through a pay-for-performance scheme that rewards them more for meeting targets based on patient satisfaction, use of evidence-based medicine and several other criteria (Elg et al., 2013).

Individual physicians are primarily salaried employees, whether in the delivery centers for primary care or in hospitals, as in the case of most specialists, although specialists may receive some per case fees as well. GPs do not function as gatekeepers for the specialists, and patients are free to self-refer to specialists. In addition to their salaries from the public health system, physicians are free to treat private patients who may be funded by private insurance. That insurance is generally supplied through employers and enables the insured to reduce waiting times for care.

Most hospitals are public and staffed by public sector employees. All these services are essentially free except for small co-pays set by the county councils (with a nationally determined limit of the annual maximum fees paid by a patient). The fees received by the delivery units for specialist care and hospitalization are based on diagnostic related groupings (DRGs) that are set at the regional level. There are also co-payments for drugs and medical appliances such as eyeglasses (depending upon need).

As was true for the United Kingdom, the Swedish healthcare system is very different from that of the United States. It is public and largely free to patients at the point of delivery, except for some small co-payments. The Swedish system is national, but also very decentralized, with county and municipal governments playing major roles in managing and funding the system. The system therefore does encounter some of the coordination problems that the even more decentralized system of the United States encounters.

France

Unlike the previous two countries discussed in this chapter, healthcare in France is an insurance-based system. Enrollment in the national health insurance program is mandatory for most citizens, and the insurance covers physicians, hospitals and long-term care. The central government regulates the provision of healthcare and allocates funds to the 17 regional health agencies that are responsible for planning and delivery of all care within their territory. Thus, the insurance scheme is itself rather centralized, while the actual delivery of health services is more decentralized.

The insurance system has been, like many social insurance programs,[5] based on employment, and was extended over the years from just covering employees to also include retirees and the self-employed. In 2000 the system was extended to cover anyone who did not fit into those employment categories. At present, all residents of France, including legal immigrants, are covered by the statutory health insurance program.

Like health insurance in the United States, the insured must make co-payments for services, and there is an opportunity for providers to "balance bill" their patients for services. That is, if the fee charged by the provider is higher than the official rate (see below) the provider can bill the patient for the difference (now up to 100 percent of the official rate). In addition to any balance billing, co-payments are substantial, for example 30 percent for out-patient doctors and dental visits. Out-of-pocket spending by citizens, however, funds only less than 7 percent of total French health expenditures. Vision and dental services are a major source of out-of-pocket payments by citizens, largely because these providers are able to balance bill significantly more than can other providers of health services.

The 7 percent figure for out-of-pocket spending does not include the spending by private, supplemental insurance that approximately 95 percent of the French public purchase. Most of this insurance is complementary and is used to fund the co-payments charged by physicians and hospitals, like Medigap insurance in the United States. Most of the private insurance is provided by employers, although the employees tend to pay at least half the total cost of the insurance. Some of the private insurance is also supplementary and covers services and products not provided through the statutory health insurance.

Most of the funding for the statutory health insurance scheme is public, coming from payroll taxes (80 percent paid by the employers), an earmarked income tax for healthcare, a tax on tobacco, pharmaceutical, and private health insurance companies, and a small amount of direct state contribution from general revenues. There are no deductibles or premiums for the public health insurance program. However, the burden of paying for the service is on the patient, who must pay the full fee and then be reimbursed, minus the co-payment. This is different from most American insurance schemes in which the patient only pays the co-pay and the insurance company pays the provider directly.[6]

GPs in France are primarily free professionals who are paid on a fee-for-service basis, although there is now some movement toward managed care, with financial incentives for patients who sign up with a physician and allow the physician to function as a gatekeeper for other healthcare services. Also, there are an increasing number of "medical homes" that provide coordinated care by several doctors, nurses and other practitioners (see Fields et al., 2010). GPs can also be paid capitation fees for managing care for patients with chronic diseases.

About one-third of all specialists are also free professionals working outside hospitals and are paid on a fee-for-service basis. Those specialists working within hospitals are salaried, or combine salaried and private employment. Self-employed specialists also must take part in a pay-for-performance program that sets targets for managing specific diseases and rewards physicians who met those targets.

The hospital sector is approximately two-thirds public, with the remainder being predominately private, for-profit facilities. Hospitals are paid for patients through a DRG system in which a single payment is made based on the diagnosis. Those fees are established by the Ministry of Social Affairs, Health, and Women's Rights. There may, however, be additional payments for especially complicated and expensive treatments, again with the rates determined by central government.

The French healthcare system is a clear example of a universal insurance-based system, with the insurance being for the most part public. That said, the relatively high co-payments required from patients have helped to create a market for private insurance that will cover those co-pays, as well as perhaps some for some supplementary services. Patients appear to have a good deal of freedom in choosing their physicians and in getting access to specialists, but issues of cost and coordination are pushing in the direction of more managed care.

Australia

The Australian healthcare system (Medicare) is a national, universal health insurance system that is administered through the states and territories. All citizens are enrolled automatically in the system, and permanent residents, New Zealanders and certain other people also can enroll. The program provides free hospital stays as well as substantial subsidies for doctors' visits, pharmaceuticals and some other services. Citizens are also encouraged to purchase private insurance that covers private hospital stays, dental care and additional services such as physical therapy, podiatry and eyeglasses. The private health insurance is subsidized through tax deductions, and the costs are regulated by government.

This health insurance scheme is funded by general revenues as well as by a Medicare Levy of 2 percent of taxable income for people who earn more than a very modest income and some individuals with reductions because of age or disability. There are also revenues from co-pays by patients for specialist services (15 percent). Physicians may also choose to charge more than the fees established by the Medicare Benefits Scheme, and those fees are paid by the patient. Although there are out-of-pocket costs for physicians' services, these expenditures have an annual limit that is partially related to income.

All three levels of government in federal Australia are involved in healthcare. The federal government is responsible for funding Medicare and regulates private insurance and most other aspects of the health system. The state level is more involved in the direct delivery of health services, most importantly public hospitals but also public dentistry. They also make some contribution to total spending for health services. Local governments provide public health services such as immunizations, and regulate some aspects of health such as food services. These various services are coordinated through a health committee of the Council of Australian Governments (COAG).

PCPs are self-employed, and are paid on a fee-for-service basis through the Medicare Benefits Scheme. The fees are set nationally, although some physicians do charge more. These GPs are also the gatekeepers of the medical care system, given that referrals are required to see specialists. Specialists are also paid on a fee-for-service basis, and approximately two-thirds are in private practice and one-third work in the public hospitals, although some split their time between the two types of practice.

The Pharmaceuticals Benefit Scheme, financed in the same way as the Medicare Benefits Scheme, subsidizes out-patient pharmaceuticals. There is a maximum out-of-pocket payment for any drug, with lower prices for individuals with lower incomes. As is true for the out-of-pocket expenditure for physicians' visits, there is a limit on the out-of-pocket expenditures for individuals each year.

The hospital sector is composed of public and private hospitals. The public hospitals receive almost all of their funding from government (federal and state), and the private hospitals receive approximately one-third of their funding from government. These hospitals are linked in local networks that coordinate services and attempt to minimize duplication of services within a local area. Given the vast geographical spaces within the country and the dispersal of the population, rural hospitals tend to be treated somewhat differently in funding to ensure that residents in those areas have accessible care.

In summary, Australia has one of the most accessible healthcare systems in the developed world. It provides universal coverage with minimal out-of-pocket expenditures for the patients. The linkage of the public system with private insurance furthers the accessibility of the system and provides additional financial support. This system is not inexpensive for government, absorbing approximately 17 percent of total spending. Adding private spending, the total amounts to over 11 percent of gross domestic product.

Germany

Like France and Australia, healthcare in Germany is insurance based, but the source of that insurance differs significantly from the other two countries. Going back to the formative stage of the welfare state in Germany, health insurance was provided through sickness funds (*Krankenkasse*) that are non-profit, competitive, organizations that work in cooperation with government to provide universal coverage. All German citizens are required to have health insurance, and approximately 85 percent have it through the statutory *Krankenkasse*. The large majority of the remaining citizens purchase insurance through private insurance funds, although there are some small schemes for certain public employees. Further, like the United Kingdom, Sweden and France, the system is universal but, unlike the others, it is delivered in large part by non-governmental actors in cooperation with public authorities.

Hospitals in Germany are approximately half public, one-third not-for-profit, and the remainder are for-profit. The for-profit segment of the mix is increasing. Hospitals are paid per admission on the basis of DRGs. The DRGs are a set of over 1,000 different diagnoses, each with a specific payment attached. The hospitals, and the salaried doctors within them, are expected to provide all necessary care for the patient for the value of the DRG. There are exceptions for highly complex diseases and procedures, but the use of DRGs is a means of controlling costs used here and elsewhere (see Chapter 3).

The health insurance system is funded through a payroll tax, half paid by employees and half by employers, although the taxes only apply to approximately the first $70,000 of earnings. The insurance fees for the unemployed and elderly are paid by government from general revenues. The coverage provided by the statutory insurance funds is regulated by the federal government through the Federal Joint Committee. The *Krankenkasse* must provide a range of basic services but are permitted to provide additional services as well, and can also compete by providing rebates for low usage. In addition, there is a separate insurance system that provides for long-term care for elderly and disabled people.

People earning more than the statutory maximum for payment into the public health funds can opt for private insurance. This insurance can be purchased from any one of several dozen companies (for-profit and not-for-profit). The premiums for these policies are generally greater than those for the statutory sickness funds, but they may provide better services. They do not, however, mean that the insured will be able to see different doctors—doctors are required to treat publicly and privately insured individuals the same.

In addition to the money received through the payroll taxes, the German health system is funded by co-payments for hospital visits, pharmaceuticals and medical appliances. These co-payments are significantly lower than those in the United States—for example, €10 a day for a hospital stay—and do not apply to some groups (children) or some services (screening). Likewise, the charges for pharmaceuticals are regulated and also significantly lower than in the United States. The co-pays still, however, constitute about 13 percent of total revenues for the German healthcare system.

GPs in the German system are free professionals who receive insurance payments on a fee-for-service basis, with the rate determined by bargaining between the *Krankenkasse* and the provider associations. Fees from private insurance are paid on top of those received from the statutory insurance system. Most specialists (other than those in hospitals) work in ambulatory care clinics containing multiple specialties, and are salaried employees of those clinics. Individuals have free choice of their doctors and, in general, access to specialists is not constrained by any gate-keeping role of the GPs.

Although there is a strong public sector role in regulating the healthcare system in Germany, much of the management and policymaking is done in a corporatist manner. For example, the Federal Joint Committee that sets the service requirements for the *Krankenkasse* is composed of representatives of the sickness funds, representatives of the providers, and three independent members. Likewise, the regional associations of physicians constitute the intermediary between the doctors and the sickness funds, and also coordinate care within the region. Although the providers are paid on a capitation basis, there are limits on the amount of billing in each quarter of the year as a cost-control mechanism. Despite the strength of corporatism in German healthcare, a number of competitive elements are being introduced in an attempt to control costs (Kifmann, 2017).

Although it has universal coverage, the German healthcare system does have some similarities with that of the United States. The delivery of health services is decentralized, and has a good deal of involvement by the private sector. It also tends to rely more on financing by co-payments than most European systems, although again not so much as the United States. Finally, the federal government is involved in the healthcare system, but utilizes a number of regulatory instruments along with more direct involvement.

Switzerland

The healthcare system of Switzerland is similar to that of Germany by being universal but highly decentralized. Indeed, it is if anything more decentralized than

Germany. The cantons in Switzerland are major actors in funding healthcare and in setting some of the healthcare policies. Also, following a long tradition of using private insurance rather than a universal model, the health insurance provided in Switzerland is closer to the private style of insurance used in the United States than is that of other European countries.

The government role in healthcare is divided among the three levels of government. The federal government's role is largely regulatory, including regulating the safety of pharmaceuticals and appliances, and it oversees public health and medical research. It also regulates the benefits that insurance schemes operated through the cantons must provide. In addition to their role in health insurance, each of the 26 cantons licenses physicians and hospitals, coordinates medical services within their territory, and subsidizes the healthcare system and individuals. The municipalities, as was true in Sweden, play a major role in long-term care and in supporting vulnerable groups in society.

Although offered by non-profit organizations analogous to the *Krankenkasse* in Germany, the insurance offered in the cantonal markets is similar to that offered in the United States. One major difference, however, is that there are no family plans; rather, each individual must have their own insurance. Individuals pay premiums for their insurance, and have choices among programs based on the amount of the annual deductible (ranging from CHF300 to CHF2,500) among other factors. In addition to the deductibles there are co-payments of 10 percent of the cost of the service or medication up to an annual maximum of CHF700 for adults or CHF350 for children. In total, the cost-sharing features of the insurance program covers roughly 5 percent of the total costs. Given that there are significant out-of-pocket costs for patients under the statutory insurance program there is also private insurance available that can cover those costs.[7]

Although much of the insurance in Switzerland is in the conventional indemnity format, there is some movement toward managed care plans in which the PCP functions as a gatekeeper and decides about referrals to specialists. Otherwise, the insured have free choice of their physicians and can refer themselves to specialists. Both primary care and specialist physicians are paid on a fee-for-service basis, with the fees being negotiated each year between the provider associations and the cantonal association (somewhat like in Germany).

The hospital sector is composed of both public and private hospitals, and includes a large number of specialized hospitals. The fees that hospitals can charge for treatment are controlled by a national DRG scheme that is determined by a national non-profit organization. This helps to contain costs and places pressures on the hospitals for efficient services. The physicians who work in the hospital sector are generally salaried, rather than working on a fee-for-service basis. The cantonal governments are responsible for coordinating hospital care, both within their own cantons and with others. This is especially important because citizens can now seek hospital care in any canton they wish. Further, some cantons or half-cantons are rather small and may not be able to support a full-service hospital.

The Swiss healthcare system appears closer to that in the United States than any of the others discussed here. That is true, despite the universality of the system. The Swiss healthcare system relies more on out-of-pocket expenditures by the insured than do the others, and the cantons have some of the same powers (as well as many more) than states in the United States have. Further, there is a significant reliance on the private sector for health insurance and some other aspects of healthcare, although the organizations involved are primarily not-for-profit.

Conclusion

I could add any number of other healthcare schemes found in other wealthy democracies, but these six cover the principal models for care, and show possible alternative models for reforming the US healthcare system. What distinguishes these cases from the United States is that they are universal, providing similar levels of access to all residents, or at least to all citizens. These systems may be decentralized in how they structure the coverage, especially in Germany, Sweden and Switzerland, but the principle of universality prevails. Although these healthcare systems are all controlled by the public sector, most also have a significant involvement of private sector actors (for-profit and/or not-for-profit).

These systems also face some common problems. One of these is cost. Although not so rapid as in the United States, costs are rising and are imposing burdens on other parts of the public budget. Most of these systems, therefore, have co-payments and perhaps deductibles to try to recover some of the costs of service and perhaps also to deter consumption. Most countries also use some form of DRGs to attempt to constrain the growth of costs within the hospital sector. Healthcare also faces the challenge of aging populations in all these countries, and with that the need to coordinate medical services with social services for the elderly and other vulnerable populations. The coordination issues also exist within the healthcare system itself, including linking primary and secondary care, linking healthcare with social care, and ensuring that all levels of government cooperate effectively.

3

Medicare: public health insurance for the elderly

The involvement of the federal government in providing health insurance to American citizens has expanded step-by-step. It has involved coverage for segments of society deemed especially deserving of protection from financial barriers to healthcare. With the exception of veterans who have received direct health services in some form since 1834, the first major involvement of the federal government was through Medicare, a health insurance program for the elderly. This program was created through amendments to the Social Security Act in 1965, as a component of President Lyndon Johnson's "Great Society" (Levitan and Taggart, 1976).

Several presidents before Johnson, going back at least to Theodore Roosevelt, had advocated some form of national health insurance, but the resistance of the American Medical Association, and the distrust of "socialized medicine" by most citizens, blocked adoption. The assassination of President John F. Kennedy opened a "policy window" for President Johnson, who had the political skills necessary to build a coalition to pass Medicare and Medicaid (see Chapter 4). This was perhaps the most important component of the Great Society program that sought to alter fundamentally levels of poverty in the United States (Marmor, 2000).

Targeting the elderly through subsidized health insurance was a very appropriate way to attack poverty at that time. Although poverty affected all age groups, it was especially prevalent among the elderly. In 1965, over 28 percent of the population over 65 lived with inadequate income to cover their expenses, and one of the major expenses was healthcare.[1] Relatively few of the elderly had health insurance—varying by region between 43 and 73 percent (Feder, 1977). Further, the elderly would be considered the "deserving poor" who were not expected to continue to work after the normal retirement age. Further, legally and politically, Medicare was treated as an extension of social security, a very popular program that had been operating for 30 years.

There had been one earlier piece of legislation that attempted to address some of these problems of the elderly. The Kerr–Mills Act created the Medical Assistance for the Aged program in 1960. This legislation did two things that would be important for subsequent legislation on healthcare. First, it recognized the special needs of the elderly for assistance with medical bills. Second, it created the concept of the "medically indigent"—those who may not be indigent in the usual sense of the term but who could not afford healthcare. This legislation became a precursor to both Medicare and Medicaid. Like Medicaid, it was delivered through the states with federal subsidies and focused on the poor, including the medically indigent.[2]

Coverage and costs

Medicare was originally designed for the elderly, but it has since been expanded to include other groups, especially disabled people. In addition, Medicare was extended to cover people suffering from end-stage renal disease (1972; see Rettig, 1991), and later individuals with amyotrophic lateral sclerosis (ALS) were added in 2001. Especially with demographic changes, the elderly represent the large majority of the recipients of the program, but the advocates for the victims of those two long-term and debilitating diseases were able to have those patients also covered through forceful lobbying.

Medicare is a very large program, the largest health insurance program (public or private) in the United States. As of 2020, there were over 52 million people enrolled in Medicare, with the number growing steadily since the inception of the program. Over 86 percent of the enrollees are eligible because of their age (Table 3.1), with the remainder being disabled or ill. Also, unlike many public sector programs, approximately 98 percent of those who are eligible for enrolling in Medicare are enrolled. This near universal enrollment is not only because of the needs of citizens for medical insurance, but also because the program is not means-tested and is conceptualized as insurance and not "welfare". People believe they have already paid for the program with their taxes and therefore are entitled to it. Given the number of people enrolled, and the costs of medical care in the United States, it is not surprising the Medicare is also a major spending program for the federal government. In 2021 Medicare expenditures totaled $889.4 billion. This was 20 percent of total health expenditures in the United States that year, which was up somewhat from the 22 percent in 2000 (see Table 3.2). This spending number does not, however, include the out-of-pocket expenditures by the insured in the form of deductibles and co-payments, so the actual economic role of Medicare is even greater.

The general opinion of most Americans is that public programs are inherently less efficient, and more bureaucratic, than are private programs. For health insurance this is not the case at all. The overhead administrative expenses of Medicare and Medicaid at the federal level[3] are approximately 2 percent of total program expenditures. This figure compares to an estimate of 14–16 percent for private

Table 3.1: Reasons for eligibility for Medicare, 2019

	Percent
Age 65 or Older	86.2
Disabled	13.7
Renal Disease	0.1
ALS	<0.1

Source: Office of Health Policy, Department of Health and Human Services, *Medicare Beneficiary Enrollment Trends*, March 2, 2022.

Table 3.2: Health consumption expenditures, 2021 (percentage of total)

Out of Pocket	10.4
Insurance	75.2
Private	27.8
Medicare	22.6
Medicaid	18.7
Other	6.1
Other Spenders and Public Health Activity	14.3

Source: Centers for Medicare and Medicaid Services, *National Health Expenditures, 2022*.

health insurance companies. The Centers for Medicare and Medicaid Services (CMS) is relatively small for the size of its budget (6,300 employees), it pays no high-priced executives and does very little paid advertising.

Financing Medicare

Given the amount of money spent by Medicare, raising sufficient revenue is an ongoing problem for the program. The fiscal pressures on Medicare are more intense because, like Social Security Part A (hospitalization), it is financed largely by an earmarked tax. Employers and employees each pay 1.45 percent of earned income as a Medicare tax, and there is an additional 0.9 percent on income over $200,000. Unlike the social security payroll tax, this tax is paid on all earned income. The payroll tax is topped-up with some money from general revenues, primarily to cover the costs of the recipients eligible because of specific diseases. Parts B and D are financed by the premiums paid by the insured for this coverage, as well as by some money from general revenue allocated by Congress.

The money received from the payroll taxes and other sources is paid into two Medicare trust funds (see Patashnik and Pateman, 2000). One is the Health Insurance Trust Fund that covers Part A, and the other is the Supplemental Medical Insurance Trust Fund that covers Parts B and D. For much of the history of the program, the income for the trust fund was greater than expenditures, so a balance accumulated. However, as the population continues to age expenditures now exceed revenues and the balance in the Health Insurance Trust Fund is now beginning to decline and will soon be exhausted (see Table 3.3). This declining balance reflects the aging population and a proportionately smaller workforce. Indeed, the specter of Medicare going "bankrupt" is raised frequently in political discourse (Lawrence, 2021), and the trustees of these funds project that the funds will run out relatively soon. The Supplemental Medical Insurance Trust Fund appears likely to remain solvent for some time, in part because it is financed by premiums and co-pays that are more likely to keep pace with increasing costs.

Table 3.3: Projections of Medicare trust fund balances ($ billions)

	Health Insurance Trust Fund	Supplemental Medical Trust Fund
2023	169.4	196.8
2024	155.1	186.7
2025	128.9	182.2
2026	93.3	192.0
2027	48.3	199.4
2028	–8.6	214.2
2029	–77.3	228.7
2030	–157.4	243.5

Source: *2022 Annual Report of Trustees of the Federal Hospital Insurance Trust Fund and the Federal Supplementary Medical Insurance Trust Funds* (Washington, DC: June 2).

The present and future problems with financing Medicare have led to a number of proposals for reforming financing. The simplest would be to remove the direct connection between the payroll tax and the program, and just finance it like any other program with general revenue. This is, however, potentially unpalatable politically given that the public appears to mind less paying taxes that are linked to specific programs. Also, the Medicare tax has been stable since 1993, except for the surtax on incomes over $200,000 added in 2013, so the tax rate might be increased to reflect the aging of the population. Also, Medicare could become means-tested, with people with higher levels of income and/or assets receiving lower rates of coverage, or paying higher premiums. There are also more extreme reforms of the entire program that will be discussed below.

Components of Medicare

Medicare is an insurance-based program. When people reach 65, or are diagnosed with one of the covered diseases, they must enroll. Even if they do not want to activate the insurance immediately (perhaps they are still covered by an employer) they need to enroll. If they do not begin to use the insurance it costs nothing; but once they do, premiums, deductible and co-payments, intended to both defray some of the total program costs and to deter consumption by the insured, will be charged. Individuals who do not enroll will have to pay penalties later if they want the insurance.

Medicare has four component programs. Parts A and B provide coverage for hospitalization and for physicians' services, and other medical services, respectively. These are both fee-for-service programs, with charges for each service rendered. Part C, or Medicare Advantage, involves private sector insurers taking fees from Medicare and then providing services to their enrollees. These programs are managed as health maintenance organizations (HMO) or preferred provider organizations (PPO), often with rather strict limits on the providers from whom the insured may receive services. In exchange, however, the insured may receive services that are not normally available through Medicare.

Part D of Medicare was added to the program as a part of the Medicare Prescription Drug Improvement and Modernization Act of 2003, and came into effect in 2006. This component was designed to address the continuing problem of the high costs of prescription medications for Medicare recipients—on average each person over the age of 65 takes over four prescription drugs every day. This part of Medicare is managed by private insurers who offer a variety of plans to Medicare participants on a state-by-state basis.

Part A

Part A of Medicare is for hospitalization and similar residential care. This part of Medicare does not require the participant to pay any premiums for coverage. However, it is far from free. As shown in Table 3.4, a patient using Part A will have to pay a considerable amount in co-pays and, if the patient has to remain in the hospital for a long period of time, the amount that they will have to pay goes up substantially. It is important to remember that this is a program designed for a population most of whom are retired and living on a fixed income. A hospital stay of even a few days will therefore easily require a month's social security income for the patient.[4]

Table 3.4: Premiums and co-pays for Medicare, 2022

Part A		
	Premiums	$0 if 40 quarters of work in covered employment.
	Hospitalization deductible	$1,556
	Co-pay for hospitalization 1–60 days	$0
	Co-pay for hospitalization 61–90 days	$389 per day
	Co-pay over 90 days	$778 per day (lifetime reserve of 60 days at that rate)
	After lifetime reserve	All costs
Part B		
	Premium	$171.10 per month or more, depending on income[1]
	Deductible	$233
	Co-pay	20% after deductible
Parts C and D		
	Premiums	Depends on plan

[1] Maximum of $578.30.

In addition to the high costs of co-pays associated with Part A, the program also provides very limited skilled nursing care for the insured. While an increasing number of elderly Americans are finding ways to remain in their homes, or finding other means for dealing with long-term care, a significant number will also spend their final years in nursing facilities. The few days covered by Medicare Part A may be totally inadequate for many elderly patients. Medicaid, the health insurance program for the medically indigent, does pay for long-term nursing care, so some patients spend their resources to be able to receive Medicaid benefits for nursing home care.

This having been said, Medicare Home Care Services do provide some support for the insured, but not extended care in nursing facilities. These services can include short-term residential care, visiting service providers, necessary medical equipment to help cope with disabilities, and physical and occupational therapy. These home services may be subject to co-pays by the recipient of the services, but using Medicare-certified providers can limit the out-of-pocket expenses. Although these services are important to the recipients, they are still not as easily available to all insured as they should be (Lyons and Rowland, 2022).

Part B

This second component of Medicare pays for physicians' services, diagnostic testing, durable medical equipment, and a number of smaller services. This part of Medicare does have premiums analogous to those in a private health insurance program (see Table 3.4). Unlike other parts of Medicare, Part B premiums are means-tested, with those earning above $91,000 per year ($182,000 for married couples filing taxes jointly) paying more. In addition to the premiums, there is a deductible before the benefits begin, and then the program pays only 80 percent of the costs. Again, for a population of beneficiaries on fixed incomes and with a large number of visits to physicians, this coverage is far from generous.

Also, just as there are some beneficiaries in the coverage provided through Part A, there are also several major problems with the coverage through Part B. For example, Medicare pays for some durable equipment, for example walkers or wheelchairs, but it does not pay for hearing aids or eyeglasses. Indeed, there is no vision coverage in Medicare, except for people with specific medical conditions such as diabetes. Hearing and vision are major problems for the elderly, and leaving those out of the program imposes even greater costs on the program beneficiaries.

Part C

The third component of Medicare was adopted in 1997 as a part of the Balanced Budget Act. This alternative, also called Medicare Advantage, within Medicare was developed as a means of reducing the costs of the program, both for government and for the beneficiary. This cost saving was to be attained by moving from a fee-for-service plan in Parts A and B to a capitation plan such as an HMO or a

PPO. For each person enrolled in a Medicare Advantage plan, a private insurer receives a flat fee that is to pay for all the services for the enrollee. The Medicare Advantage plans may also add other services not normally covered by Parts A and B, and compete with one another by offering things such as vision and dental services (see Pope, 2016). These plans can also charge deductibles and co-pays up to $6,700 per year, although many advertise not having any such fees.

To be able to provide those extra benefits, Medicare Advantage plans must save money elsewhere. The HMOs used to deliver the services may place a number of restrictions on the patients. Patients may encounter more difficulties in seeing specialists, perhaps requiring prior authorization, which conventional Medicare does not have, and they may have a narrow network of physicians and facilities that they can use. The formulary for drugs may also be more restrictive, so that patients may not be able to get the exact drugs their physician may prefer. Thus, the patients may pay for their extra benefits with some inconveniences in other aspects of their care. Despite those restrictions, there is some evidence that the quality of healthcare is at least as good in Medicare Advantage as it is in fee-for-service Medicare, especially after quality bonuses were added as an incentive for the Part C providers during the Obama administration (KFF, 2011; but see Grimm, 2022).

The financing of Medicare Part C has been a continuing issue for the program. As already noted, the initial plan was for Part C to reduce Medicare costs by up to 5 percent (McGuire et al., 2011). Over time the results have turned out to be exactly the opposite, with Medicare Advantage now costing on average more than conventional Medicare. The difference between payments for Part C and conventional Medicare was reduced in part by the Affordable Care Act (Kapstan, 2011). The program has, to some extent, become a subsidy to private insurers who may offer their insured some additional benefits, but with the additional costs being paid largely by government. These costs are likely to increase, given that enrollment in Part C has increased significantly and the projections are that it will increase to 61 percent of Medicare beneficiaries by 2032 (Freed et al., 2022). Also, there have been a number of issues raised about the private insurers overcharging Medicare (Abelson and Sanger-Katz, 2023).

Part D

Even more than Part C, Medicare Part D illustrates the "jungle" nature of American healthcare. This component of Medicare was adopted by the George W. Bush administration to attempt to solve the enduring problem of high drug prices for senior citizens. When passed, the legislation missed an opportunity to use the market power of the federal government to lower drug prices. Not surprisingly, perhaps, one of the architects of the legislation soon left Congress after its passage to become an executive at a major pharmaceutical industry lobbying organization (Slaughter, 2006).

The plan that was created was extremely complex, and baffled many recipients. In addition, there were multiple possible providers from which patients had to choose, each offering somewhat different services and access to drugs. For example, were I to sign up for Part D I would face a choice among almost 30 possible plans where I live in Pennsylvania, and different areas of the country will have different options. These multiple plans mean that the same drug may cost different patients very different amounts, and the amount may also depend upon which pharmacy they choose to use (Maas, 2022).

Individuals who enroll in a Part D program must first pay an annual premium. That amount depends on the plan, and the individual must therefore compare costs and benefits among all the available plans. In addition to the premium, higher income individuals have to pay an "Income Related Monthly Adjustment Account", with the maximum being $77.90 per month for individuals with incomes over $500,000 ($750,000 for married couples filing jointly). The premium is, however, only the beginning of the charges. The next charge is the deductible, or the amount that the insured must spend out-of-pocket before insurance begins to pay part of the costs of drugs. Each program will have a different deductible, with the maximum being $480 per year. Some policies charge nothing.

After the annual deductible has been paid, for all Part D programs the plan begins to pay a certain percentage of the costs of each prescription drug, with the percentage of co-payment depending on the plan purchased. When the insured and the plan together have paid a total of $4,430 (2022) then the insured will pay a maximum of 25 percent for drugs until they have paid $7,050.[5] After having paid that $7,050 the insured enters "catastrophic coverage" and will only have to pay a very small co-payment of 5 percent for drugs for the rest of the year. The current arrangements, although somewhat complex, are actually simpler than Part D was prior to reforms in the Affordable Care Act and some implemented by the Trump administration (see Sachs, 2021).

Prescription medications are expensive in the United States, and Medicare Part D does help with those expenses. That said, however, the individual still must pay several thousand dollars if they are taking several prescription drugs. This is in addition to the money already paid for Part B. For senior citizens on a fixed income these expenditures amount to a significant portion of their income. Medicare has done a great deal of good in improving the health status and economic well-being of senior citizens, but the program still imposes high costs on its insured.

Medigap insurance

Although it is not really a part of Medicare, the private insurance industry offers a large array of "Medigap" policies that cover at least part of the deductibles and co-payments charged by Medicare. These policies may also provide some coverage for vision and hearing services, and other services covered inadequately or not at all by Medicare. The out-of-pocket expenses associated with Medicare are significant, and approximately two-thirds of Medicare insured also purchase Medigap insurance. There is a large and competitive market for Medigap insurance, and those Medicare recipients with the highest probabilities of using a large amount of healthcare services, that is the very elderly and those with chronic conditions, appear, rather logically, to be more likely to purchase the insurance.

While Medigap insurance does tend to reduce out-of-pocket expenditures for the insured, it may have the unintended effect of increasing total spending on healthcare (Keane and Stavrunova, 2016). If an individual has paid for the additional insurance, in addition to having already paid for Medicare, he or she may feel that they should recoup some of their investment by utilizing more healthcare. This rather perverse incentive is a problem for any type of insurance in a fee-for-service medical system, but it is especially important for the elderly on Medicare who have on average more medical needs.

Long-term care insurance is another form of insurance that covers some of the holes in Medicare coverage. As mentioned previously, Medicare does not cover extensive stays in skilled nursing facilities, but a very large number of Americans will spend at least some part of their final years in such facilities. Individuals facing an extended period in a nursing home do have the option of spending down their resources so that they become eligible for Medicaid, which does cover nursing home care, but many prefer to buy insurance. This insurance is not inexpensive, often generally costing $300–400 a month for a policy that will pay around $300,000. That is slightly less than the current cost of three years in a nursing home. Again, this gap in coverage by Medicare represents a major financial problem for senior citizens.

Subsidies for low-income recipients

Medicare is an insurance program for which individuals are eligible based on age or having some dread disease. It is not a means-tested program like many other social programs, including Medicaid. That said, given that the premiums, co-pays and deductibles included in Medicare can be a major burden on the less affluent elderly, there is a need to take the financial situations of the insured into account. Therefore, the states are empowered to provide subsidies to patients who meet certain income criteria, usually based on the federal poverty level. In many states individuals may be disqualified from receiving these subsidies if they have significant assets. For example, in Arkansas a couple can have no more than $11,100 in assets if they want to receive assistance, while in neighboring Louisiana there is no limit on the assets of people receiving low-income assistance.

Although more than ten million insured are enrolled in one or another Medicare subsidy, these differences among the states emphasize the "jungle" nature of American healthcare (see Chapter 1). Although Medicare is a federal program and for the most part is managed directly by the federal government, the capacity of people to take part in the program, or to take part in it without excessive financial burdens, may depend on where they live. Only 7 percent of Medicare beneficiaries in North Dakota are enrolled in a subsidy program, while 33 percent of those in the District of Columbia receive the subsidies (KFF, 2022b). The barriers may be especially high for Part D (prescription drugs) given the very high costs of some pharmaceuticals in the United States, and the number of medications that the average senior citizen must take each day.

Politics of Medicare

Medicare is one of the most popular programs in the federal government. Along with its fellow social insurance program, Social Security, more Americans tend to support this program than they do others (see Table 3.5). The logic of this support is rather obvious. If they are not themselves one of the almost 70 million recipients of benefits, they almost certainly have a parent or a grandparent who is. Further, they may look forward to receiving these benefits once they reach 65 years of age, and want the program to remain in place for them. This widespread support exists despite some of the discussed deficiencies of the program.

Medicare is also supported because it has worked. The health status of older Americans, and their life expectancy, has been improved in part due to this program. It may be impossible to determine how much of that improvement is due to Medicare and how much is due to general improvements in healthcare, better diet, etc., but certainly Medicare has contributed. Further, a much smaller proportion of the population is now living in poverty because a good portion of their medical expenses are now covered by this insurance.

Privatization

One of the continuing political issues for Medicare is its possible privatization. Almost from its inception, the extremely large costs of the program for the federal government have led many politicians to advocate reducing costs through private sector solutions. As argued above, competition has not always been effective as a mechanism for cost control in healthcare, but the free-market assumptions that

Table 3.5: Relative importance of federal government programs (percent saying "very important")

Social Security	83
Medicare	77
Aid to Education	75
Defense	73
College Student Loans	64
Medicaid	63
Foreign Aid	18

Source: Kaiser Family Foundation, *Poll*, 2019.

dominate American policymaking still led to calls for privatization of some or all of the program.

Part C of Medicare is already a privatized delivery program for the benefits that might ordinarily be delivered through Parts A and B. Private insurance companies provide Part C benefits through contracts with HMOs and other providers, and make a profit doing so. These programs have been popular with many participants because of the expanded benefits that are provided, and they do appear to have saved government some money, at least initially. Those savings, however, may arise from the use of managed care rather than from private provision itself.

Although Part C has been successful, other attempts to privatize the program have been met with strong opposition. The most notable attempt to privatize Medicare was made by President George W. Bush. This was an important plank in his campaign for the presidency in 2000. Then, as a part of the Medicare Modernization Act of 2003—the legislation that also created Part D—there was a large increase in the amount of support given to the private firms that provided Medicare Advantage plans by removing caps that had been put into place by the Balanced Budget Act. In advocating these changes, President Bush stressed the importance of increased competition to providing better service to the public (Oberlander, 2007).

There was a second major attempt to privatize Medicare during the Trump administration. This modification of the program was called "Direct Contracting". The idea for direct contracting is that, like Medicare Advantage, a private entity would manage the medical care of the recipients. That entity would be a middleman between the CMS and the insured. In the extreme version of this plan, based on geography, a contractor would become responsible for managing all Medicare fee-for-service patients in its territory. They would be managed essentially as a PPO, which presumably would save money.

The privatization of Medicare, or at least a significant downsizing of the program, has arisen again in Congress in 2023. One segment of the new Republican majority in the House of Representatives has advocated cutting Medicare (and social security) spending, given that the trust funds are in danger of being exhausted. These proposals have been extremely vague by the time of this writing, but may pose yet another challenge to the program that is both popular and very expensive.

Another option for organizing Medicare services has been suggested. This would be the accountable care organizations (ACOs) created as a part of the Affordable Care Act. These ACOs are in essence HMOs that would receive a flat payment each year from CMS for each patient and would be expected to provide all the healthcare services required. If this annual fee is set correctly then the ACO could at least break even, and CMS may be able to save some money as well. Finding this optimal level of funding is, however, difficult given the patient mix (how many very old patients, for example) and the possibility of outbreaks of contagious diseases, and many other contingencies.

For both the Bush and Trump administrations, any direct efforts to privatize Medicare were unsuccessful, and politically unpopular. Very much like opposition to efforts to privatize social security, the public appears to have become accustomed to having a public health insurance program for the elderly, and does not want to take any chances with radical changes. Most citizens depend on the program to take care of an aging family member, and they want the program there for them when they reach age 65.

Public opinion and Medicare

Part of the reason for the difficulties in privatizing Medicare is that it is very popular with the public. Indeed, it is among the most popular of all programs in the federal government—the only program that citizens want more increases in spending in is education. Twice as many respondents wanted to decrease spending for national defense as wanted to decrease spending on Medicare. Likewise, only Social Security is considered to be a more important program than Medicare (Table 3.5). This positive ranking reflects the importance of the program to such a large segment of the population, and the potential relevance for the entire population.

Although the public generally supports Medicare, there is a good deal of skepticism about the future of the program. The talk of bankruptcy of the program has made many people concerned about whether the program will still exist when they are ready to take part in it. For example, in 2009 three-quarters of the population thought Medicare was in a fiscal crisis and, although that proportion dropped to six in ten in 2014, the perception of the future was not positive (Brodie, et al., 2015). This skepticism is especially pronounced among younger people, who do not think they will receive benefits, or at least not full benefits, from the program, even though they may already be paying Medicare taxes as they work.[6] Perhaps because of their skepticism about the future of the program, and despite the perceptions of importance, the public are not very satisfied with Medicare and Social Security. Unfortunately, this sequence of surveys over a number of years does not differentiate opinions about the two programs. They are closely linked, but it is still possible for someone to like one and dislike the other. Whether the stability should be considered a positive or a negative is unclear, but the level of discontent with Medicare and social security has been relatively persistent over time.

Medicare reform

While privatization does not appear to be a welcome change within Medicare, other less drastic reforms might be possible. These reforms could preserve the essence of the program while providing enough cost-savings, or additional revenues, to enable the program to survive. Further, as pointed out in this chapter, the benefits provided through Medicare are far from outstanding, so other reforms might expand benefits such as vision care, or nursing home care; but those changes would in turn add to the costs of the program and further threaten its survival.

Table 3.6: Evaluations of Medicare and Social Security

	Very Satisfied	Somewhat Satisfied	Somewhat Dissatisfied	Very Dissatisfied	No Answer
2022	12	26	25	29	9
2020	12	33	25	22	6
2018	11	32	25	25	7
2016	8	32	28	27	5
2014	12	30	25	25	6
2012	9	25	28	32	7
2008	8	23	29	35	5
2005	8	23	29	36	4
2001	6	32	32	25	5

Source: Gallup, *In-Depth Topics*, https://news.gallup.com/poll/14596/medicare.aspx.

A first set of reforms would be to find new sources of revenue for Medicare so that it can continue to function as it does now. The simplest reform of this sort would be to pay for Medicare from general taxation, for example income tax revenue. This would, however, break the link between an earmarked tax and the benefit that has been part of the political justification of the program, and might make the program more subject to attacks by conservatives. Some more extreme conservatives are already expressing a desire to end Medicare as an entitlement (Wang, 2022). Even if the payroll tax continued to be collected and any deficit was made up by general taxation, the tradition of social insurance programs being just that—insurance—might be threatened.

A second option would be to add yet another tax, or replace the payroll tax with another tax. The usual candidate for a new tax is the value-added tax (VAT) as is implemented in most European countries (Long and Smeeding, 1984). In this case the value-added tax would become a national sales tax that would either supplement existing revenues or replace the current tax.[7] No politician wants to advocate a new tax, especially in the United States, and the VAT has been opposed by many critics as being a "stealth tax" that would not be obvious to the taxpayer and therefore could easily be increased.

A final source of revenue could come from increasing the additional income-related premiums that the more affluent must pay. Already the insured who earn over $500,000 a year must pay over $7,000 more each year for coverage in Parts B and D combined. While this may not be appear to be a huge amount to someone with that level of income, the amount that is being paid might be as much or more than they would pay for private insurance, with perhaps better coverage. Raising these income-related payments might therefore have the effect of actually reducing total income for the program.

If the finances of Medicare cannot be improved by increasing revenues, then perhaps they can be improved by reducing expenditures. We know (see Chapter 9) that there is a great deal of fraud and waste in Medicare spending. Exercising more effective oversight over expenditures and reimbursements could (were controls bordering on perfect) perhaps reduce current spending by up to 10 percent. That could certainly help to keep the program going for some time, but would not be a long-term solution, given continuing demographic changes.

Medicare could also benefit greatly from a general reduction in drug prices, given the amount of money that is spent on prescription medications by the insured. Medicare is forbidden by law from negotiating drug prices with manufacturers, although the tremendous market power of this number of insured would be able to produce very large discounts. The states that administer Medicaid have no such restriction and are able to save billions of dollars. The political power of the pharmaceutical industry in Washington—"Big Pharma"—makes any major change in this provision unlikely, but it would be the route to very large savings (Kesselheim et al., 2021).

Some of the expenditure control being sought through privatization could be attained using organizational means such as HMOs and PPOs managed directly through Medicare. By having a flat annual fee for each member of an HMO the costs for the program are more predictable, and likely less than in the existing fee-for-service program. If these structures could be managed by health delivery organizations such as hospitals rather than a private entity such as an insurance company then the benefits could be realized more easily.

Table 3.7 shows public evaluations of a number of alternatives for addressing the financial problems of Medicare. The most popular option is allowing Medicare to negotiate with drug companies (see Chapter 8), and there is substantial support for a number of other ways to reduce expenditures or increase revenues. What the respondents did not want, however, was to increase the premiums being charged to the insured.

The bulk of the discussion of reform in Medicare has been about balancing the books but, as important as that is, there is a bigger question of whether the program needs to provide expanded services to the insured. As discussed above, Medicare

Table 3.7: Support for proposals to reduce funding deficit in Medicare (percent supporting)

	Total	Over 65 years of age
Require Companies to Negotiate Drug Prices	85	83
Increase Premiums for High Income Seniors	59	56
Raise Eligibility to 67	48	64
Reduce Payments to Hospitals	46	35
Increase Payroll Taxes	43	44
Increase Premiums	13	17

Source: Kaiser Family Foundation, *Poll*, January 2013.

does not provide some services that appear especially important for senior citizens. Perhaps the most important of the holes in the program is coverage for long-term care, a service that will be needed by much of a population that will likely be living into their 80s and 90s. In addition, adding vision and hearing services would be a major benefit to the insured in this age group. The question, however, is how to pay for it all, as valuable as those services would be for the elderly.

Most of the reforms discussed for Medicare are focused on the costs to government and to citizens. However, Medicare (and Medicaid) cannot provide services if there are no physicians and hospitals that will accept this insurance. The public health insurance programs pay lower rates to physicians and other providers than do private health insurance companies. These differentials are especially noticeable in high-cost, urban areas. Of course, reforming Medicare to provide for higher fees will cost more money that will have to be provided by the insured, by taxpayers, or a combination of the two.

The Affordable Care Act (passed in 2010) made some limited attempts to improve the financial condition of Medicare. One of the goals of the legislation was to move Medicare away from fee-for-service toward more managed care, and greater integration of care among various providers. This goal led to a reduction in some Medicare reimbursements and, simultaneously, the development of incentives for value-based medicine that would both lower overall costs and improve quality (LaPointe, 2016).

Finally, although it is not necessarily a reform within the Medicare program per se, the program could benefit significantly from stronger linkages with social programs. For example, many elderly people may have surgery and then be discharged from hospital. They have no family living nearby and are not recovered sufficiently to take care of themselves adequately and safely. The result is that they are back in hospital soon after their release. What is needed in many cases is not skilled nursing care, but rather some social supports at home. The program is slowly evolving to provide that type of service, but has a very long way to go to meet the needs of many elderly patients.

Also, reform of Medicare could be considered in the context of total medical costs in the economy. Raising the age for eligibility might save Medicare some money, but lowering the age to 60, as mentioned by President Biden, could save healthcare spending in total. This result is simply because the reimbursement rates for Medicare are lower than for most private insurance policies (Lopez et al., 2020) This shift in responsibility would be another example of the piecemeal reform in healthcare that have had the federal government slowly become more involved over recent decades in healthcare.

Conclusion

The adoption of Medicare, along with Medicaid, was a major milestone in the healthcare system of the United States. It was the first significant move in what has been a piecemeal increase in the role of the federal government in providing health insurance to citizens. Medicare has had the effect of improving the economic standing of senior Americans, as well as improving their health status. Despite a number of weaknesses in the program, notably the absence of coverage for long-term care, the program is largely seen as a success. It is so much of a success that a significant portion of the American public would like to extend the program to the entire population.

The program has evolved from the time at which it was adopted to the present. When first adopted, it looked more like a standard health insurance policy for the elderly than it now does. Financial pressures have converted universal premiums to means-related premiums. Political pressures have added new groups of beneficiaries, and also added supports for less affluent elderly. Other political pressures have involved the private sector in what began as an entirely public program. In short, the jungle aspect of Medicare has increased, and may continue to increase.

Even if Medicare is not extended to cover the entire population, it will face challenges. The financing of the program is increasingly strained as the population continues to age, and new medications, perhaps especially those for Alzheimer's disease, impose extremely high costs. The financial pressures, as well as conservative ideology, are making privatization a more acceptable option for many decision-makers. That change may undermine the choice available to the insured (assuming they can find physicians willing to provide services) as well as move American healthcare further away from full public insurance.

4

Medicaid and CHIP: medical care for the medically indigent

Medicaid was adopted in the same legislation as adopted Medicare. Rather than targeting a population based on age, Medicaid was directed at people who were generally incapable of paying for health insurance on their own, and who did not receive insurance through their employers. Given the costs of health insurance in the United States, there was a significant number of people in the country who needed this type of support. Even more than Medicare, which was providing insurance to the "worthy" group of elderly Americans, the adoption of this program was perhaps only possible when the "policy window" (Kingdon, 2003) opened during the time of the Great Society, and the connection to Medicare.

The second program discussed in this chapter—the Children's Health Insurance Program (CHIP)—is, like Medicare, age-related. The program is targeted to children whose parents were too affluent to be eligible for Medicaid, but yet could not provide adequate health insurance for their children. CHIP was adopted in 1997, during what is now considered a rare moment of bipartisan policy development. As was true for Medicare, this program provided health insurance for a segment of society that even most conservatives would accept as worthy of public protection and, unlike most policies, maintained general bipartisan support for some time (Iglehart, 2007).

Both Medicaid and CHIP are administered by the states, rather than directly by the federal government. This choice was in part a recognition of the long-standing role of the states in providing medical care for the indigent. Louisiana, for example, had a "charity hospital" system throughout the state that had for decades been providing indigent care, and many other states had some sort of provision of medical care for those who could not afford it. Likewise, the Kerr–Mills legislation that preceded Medicaid (see Chapter 3) was implemented through the states. This mechanism for delivering the services also leveraged state money to help pay for the services. Although the program is implemented by the states, Medicaid is heavily regulated by the federal government, through the Centers for Medicare and Medicaid Services, but the state basis of administration does allow individual states to put some of their own stamp on the program. The capacity to adapt the program to the health, and political, needs of the states is facilitated by the existence of waiver options (Schneider, 1997).

Medicaid

Medicaid is a very large program for the states and for the federal government. Toward the end of 2021 there were almost 78 million people with health insurance through this program. This constituted approximately 18 percent of the American population. In addition to the large population covered, the program is a major spending program. In 2021 combined federal and state spending on Medicaid was $613 billion, which is approximately three-quarters of the amount spent on Medicare. As will be discussed in more detail later, the Affordable Care Act has expanded Medicaid access in most states, and helped to reduce even further the number of uninsured persons in the country.

Eligibility for Medicaid

Medicaid is designed for individuals who have insufficient income to be able to purchase medical insurance if it is not provided by their employer. Although there are some general criteria for eligibility set by the federal government, each state determines eligibility for its own program. One major issue in eligibility is whether single adults, or even couples without children, are eligible. A number of states in the South and Midwest deny Medicaid to single adults other than disabled people and pregnant women, making Medicaid analogous to several other social programs directed toward families and children. This stipulation also tends to make Medicaid appear more like a welfare program than a health insurance program.

Eligibility for Medicaid is based on the percentage of the official poverty level that the potential recipient has as income. Federal requirements are that families with children with 138 percent of the poverty level or less income are eligible. In most states that have expanded Medicaid in response to the Affordable Care Act (see below), individuals, with 138 percent or less of the poverty level, are also eligible. In some Southern and Midwestern states the income criteria for individuals are extremely restrictive—Texas provides Medicaid only to individuals with 14 percent of the poverty level or less, which in turn means it has the lowest level of health insurance coverage of any state.

Medicaid is also available to pregnant women who meet the family income levels for eligibility, and in many states the income levels are even higher. For example, in Texas the eligibility level for pregnant women is 198 percent of the poverty level. This coverage has been important in reducing levels of infant mortality and maternal mortality, although these statistics remain higher in the United States than in other consolidated democracies.

In 2022 the American Rescue Plan passed by the Biden administration gave states the option of extending coverage of Medicaid for women who had given birth for a full year after the birth. Prior to this option the standard was 60 days of coverage. The federal government will support this option for at least five years. The evidence was that there were a number of post-partum medical problems that impacted these women; maternal mortality in the United States is also very high. The extended coverage would improve the health status for the mothers and for their children, and would save lives (see Daw et al., 2021). As of mid-July, 2022 34 states had adopted, or were in the process of adopting, this extension, and another two states had implemented a partial adoption of the plan. The states that did not extend coverage were almost entirely in the upper-Midwest or the mountain west (KFF, 2022a; Stolberg, 2022).

The level of income of the potential beneficiary is not the only criterion for eligibility for Medicaid. In addition, disability is an important criterion for eligibility, especially receiving benefits from the Social Security Disability program. In addition, as noted, pregnant women are eligible for Medicaid if they have no other insurance, as are some elderly. The capacity to receive Medicaid benefits is very important for the elderly given that Medicare does not provide coverage for long-term nursing care, or for medical appliances such as hearing aids, while Medicaid does provide that coverage.

The states have another option if they want to make more of their citizens eligible for Medicaid. Federal law allows states not to count certain types of income that might put a family over the threshold of eligibility. For example, in some states veteran's pensions are not counted as income. That said, some states, for example California and Hawaii, which have very liberal rules for income for the elderly who want Medicaid benefits in order to pay for nursing home care, require that the recipients use almost all income they may have to pay for the care, with Medicaid covering the remainder. In addition, some states permit Medicaid to recover costs from the estates of individuals who have died (Leys, 2023).

The eligibility question became more significant with the passage of the Affordable Care Act in 2010. The Act provided federal money to expand eligibility for Medicaid, and initially mandated that expansion. The Supreme Court declared that this mandate was unconstitutional (see Chapter 5), but states were still permitted to choose to expand eligibility with federal support. Some 29 states decided to extend Medicare coverage almost immediately, with a number of Southern and Midwestern states opting out. Since that time, a number of those who opted out of the program initially have chosen to expand coverage. Several of these extensions have come through referendums that overturned decisions by elected officials not to extend the program to people with higher incomes. These have occurred in heavily Republican states, and the success of those referendums is indicative of the popularity of the Medicaid program, as well as a general recognition of the importance of medical insurance for all citizens.

Medicaid services

Although having its own complexities, Medicaid is a less complex program than Medicare. Medicaid insurance provides the usual coverages required to enable the insured to consume medical care. Those insured by Medicaid have access to physicians, hospitalization and rehabilitation services. Also, unlike Medicare, it also provides some coverage for hearing and vision, as well as limited dental services for individuals under 21. The states can add dental care for adults, and all but three have added at least emergency services. Perhaps most importantly, Medicaid provides long-term care in nursing homes, a service that is crucial for the elderly that is not provided by Medicare (Ng et al., 2010). In 2021 over 60 percent of all residents in long-term care facilities were insured by Medicaid.

Medicaid began as a fee-for-service program like much of American medicine, but in over half the states the program has been converted to managed care plans. This move has reduced total expenditures and also has reduced administrative expenditures (Gold et al., 1996). While that form of healthcare delivery does save money, it is not clear that it also can deliver the same quality of care. For example, managed care tends to be associated with more fragmented care, with the patient not seeing the same doctor on a regular basis, and that can be related to poorer outcomes (Kern et al., 2020).

Although Medicaid is directed toward less affluent citizens, in many states there are still some co-payments required for services. These co-payments are not required for some classes of Medicaid enrollees, such as pregnant women and children receiving preventative care. Likewise, co-pays are not charged for emergency care or for family-planning services. As is true for out-of-pocket expenses in general in American health services, the co-payments and deductibles for Medicaid have been tending to increase, both in amount and in the number of states that employ them. While the fees charged may appear nominal to more affluent people, for the Medicaid population they are often enough to deter consumption, which may have longer-term consequences for the health of the individuals (and for the overall costs of the program).

The politics of Medicaid

The politics of Medicaid are more contentious than the politics associated with Medicare. This is first because it is a means-tested program providing benefits to individuals who cannot pay for medical care themselves. For conservatives, the assumption has been that these people should simply work more to be able to pay their own way. Although the program has been in existence for almost 60 years, it is still disliked by many politicians and many citizens who do not want to pay taxes to support medical services for this relatively poor population.

Although there has been opposition from conservatives to the Medicaid program, many of the states were in favor of the program. The states were already paying a good deal of money for medical care for the indigent and the elderly and, given the demographic and economic trends, the states could identify major stresses emerging in their budgets. Therefore, state governments were generally willing to involve the federal government in a function that historically had been dominated by the states. Since the program has been initiated the states have become polarized over Medicaid, along with many other aspects of political life in the United States. More liberal states have expanded the program and made greater use of its potential, while more conservative states have sought to limit eligibility and impose work requirements.

Issues of race also often are involved in the politics of Medicaid, although for the most part erroneously. It has been argued that the decision creating separate Medicare and Medicaid programs in 1965 was shaped by racial concerns, and the assumption that most Medicaid recipients would be Black. Although many people continue to assume that most recipients of Medicaid insurance are Black or Hispanic, the largest single group of insured are white, and a significant proportion are white residents of rural areas. Thus, the largest single group of recipients of Medicaid are similar demographically to the average Trump voter in 2016 and 2020. Despite that reality, the resistance to Medicaid often has racial overtones, including among physicians (Greene at al., 2006; Emerson, 2022).

Federalism and Medicaid

The delivery of Medicaid services through state governments demonstrates the importance of federalism in American public policy. The federal government is the major funder for the program, but state governments have the opportunity to make many decisions about the details (and therefore the costs) of Medicaid. As already noted, the states may choose to add programs to the minimum required. One of the most important of these additions is contraception, which is covered in only 21 states.[1] In addition, the states can also make choices about whether to move away from traditional fee-for-service to managed care.

Medicaid represents a very large proportion of spending by the states. In 2021 approximately one tax dollar in five raised by state governments goes to Medicaid, and when the federal contribution is added the program constitutes roughly a quarter of state spending. The federal grant for Medicaid is essentially a categorical grant, dedicated to this one purpose, although there have been pressures to convert it to a block grant that would also cover other health purposes, giving the states greater autonomy. The federal grant covers at least 50 percent of Medicaid spending in the states, with poorer states receiving a higher proportion of their spending—the highest (Mississippi) receiving 78 percent. In addition to the basic formula for funding, there are additional funds available for hospitals with a large number of Medicaid recipients, as well as some additional funds that encourage quality improvements and enhance services for rural and especially impoverished constituencies.

Block granting

One of the major proposed reforms of Medicaid during the Trump administration was to move Medicaid to a block grant program that rolls up all, or at least most, federal support for health programs at the state level in a single block grant. This change in the type of grants would then permit the states to make their own decisions about how to spend the money, rather than having to conform to federal restrictions. In addition to the capacity of the states to move money around within the general health policy domain, the block grant would not be the open-ended commitment that the Medicaid program is for the federal government.

The proposal from the Trump administration was not the first time block granting for Medicaid had been proposed—this has been a common proposal from Republican politicians. The administration of George W. Bush, for example, pushed for this type of reform, as well as attempting to privatize some aspects of Medicare. Also, at the very end of the Trump administration it issued a waiver to Tennessee to allow a block grant, which has subsequently been repealed by the Biden administration (Sanger-Katz, 2021).

The benefits for the federal government of reducing expenditure liability are to some extent offset by the potential liabilities that this change in funding would create for the states. The states would place themselves in the position of being responsible for any surge in health expenditures, for example during a pandemic. Given that state revenues tend to be less buoyant than federal revenues, this could pose major problems for the state government, so that they may have to reduce eligibility or levels of reimbursement (Miller, 2014). Further, recent experience shows that, left to themselves, many states—almost all dominated by Republicans—would reduce eligibility for Medicaid, or impose harsh behavioral requirements on recipients.

The proposal for block granting in the Trump administration, called the Healthy Adult Opportunity initiative, was directed at reducing expenditures—despite the more positive name of the program. The idea was to allow the states to develop demonstration programs for services for non-disabled adults under 65 that could save money. The states would agree to an expenditure cap, and could retain a part of the federal grant if their expenditures were less than the cap. In return for accepting the cap, the states would be given great latitude in imposing restrictions on the use of the program, thus cutting services to the insured (Rudowitz et al., 2020).

Waivers

One of the most important aspects of the federal nature of Medicaid is the capacity of the states to apply for waivers from the standard requirements imposed by the federal government. These waivers are intended to permit the states to experiment and to innovate with the way in which Medicaid is delivered, but the effects on the program recipients are not always as positive as the waiver program was originally intended to be. Many of the waivers in recent years have been to impose additional requirements, including working requirements, on potential recipients. In a number of other cases waivers have been used to move toward managed care rather than fee-for-service provision for Medicaid recipients.

States can apply to the Department of Health and Human Services (HHS) for so-called 1115 waivers.[2] The Secretary of HHS is formally authorized to grant the waivers, but much of the decision actually rests with the Centers for Medicare and Medicaid Services. The Trump plan for block granting, for example, was conceived as a waiver for states that sought to gain greater control over the types of spending for Medicaid. Waivers have been used for a variety of experiments in service delivery. For example, Alabama has applied for 15 waivers since the beginning of Medicaid—all but one approved—that ranged from programs to make healthcare more community based to attempts to impose work requirements on recipients.

The changes in the program through waivers, as well as differences in eligibility requirements, co-payments, and other aspects of the program that are optional, mean that there are significant differences among the states. A Medicaid recipient in California, for example, is markedly better served than one in most Southern states. Even in states that appear to have more generous Medicaid programs, there are often exclusions of different diseases in the various states. Federalism gives state governments many options for adjusting programs to suit their political preferences, but those differences may well not suit the preferences of their citizens on the program.

Medicaid and COVID-19

COVID-19 had a major impact on the medical system of the United States (and every other country). While the pandemic did not respect the income of individuals, lower income citizens in the United States have borne a disproportionate burden of the disease. For Medicaid recipients there was a particular problem because of the large number of Medicaid recipients in nursing homes and other extended care facilities. The large number of vulnerable people living in these facilities made them a clear opportunity for the rapid transmission of the disease (Ouslander and Grabowski, 2020).

The Families First Coronavirus Recovery Act, passed early in the crisis caused by the pandemic, was an attempt to address some of the costs of COVID-19 (Clemens et al., 2021). Among other things, the Act required states to maintain enrollment of current recipients of Medicaid until the end of the public health emergency. In addition, the Act provided additional funds—an increase of 6.2 percent to federal matching funds—to the states to cover the additional costs of the program resulting from a larger enrollment.

When the pandemic began to wind down in 2022 there was the potential for over 16 million current recipients to lose coverage (Rosenthal, 2022). When the public health emergency is over, states will no longer have to maintain enrollment and can begin to remove people from Medicaid who, for whatever reason, are no longer eligible. Even for those who may be able to remain covered by this insurance, there will be substantial uncertainty, even though they will have a grace period of coverage once they are deemed ineligible. For the states, determining eligibility will be a major administrative burden. That administrative burden will be no less significant for the citizens who may have to prove their eligibility (Kelman, 2022). The Omnibus Spending Bill passed at the very end of 2022 contained a number of incentives for the states to maintain expanded Medicaid coverage after the public health emergency ends (LaFraniere and Weiland, 2023; Sanger-Katz, 2023).

CHIP

The Children's Health Insurance Program (CHIP) was adopted in 1997 during the Clinton Administration. The legislation was part of the Balanced Budget Act, and emerged as a response to the failure of President Clinton's proposal for a national health insurance program. This was an age in which Congress still worked in a bipartisan manner, and the sponsors of CHIP (originally SCHIP—State Child Health Insurance Program) were senators Ted Kennedy (D-MA) and Orrin Hatch (R-UT). This coalition of one of the most liberal and one of the most conservative senators indicates the capacity that programs serving children have to be adopted in a political system that has been a welfare state laggard.

CHIP is designed to provide health insurance to children up to age 16 whose parents are ineligible for Medicaid but who cannot afford insurance. These are the "working poor" who have some regular income but whose employers do not provide health insurance as a benefit of employment or, if they do, the premiums paid by the employees are too high for many of the employees.[3] However, like Medicaid there are income limits for families to receive CHIP insurance, usually 200 percent of the federal poverty level. Given that more employers are dropping coverage for dependents, or dropping health insurance for their employees entirely, the number of uninsured children has begun to increase again.

The children of the working poor are not the only recipients of health insurance through CHIP. Eligibility in some states has been extended to cover pregnant women, with the logic that the health of the mother is crucial for the health of the child. Over time eligibility in some states has been extended to the parents of covered children, so that in those states CHIP has become de facto family health insurance. The administration of George W. Bush sought to reduce the growth of CHIP, but the Obama administration that followed promoted the extension of the program, along with its own Affordable Care Act (see Chapter 5).

The federal expenditure for CHIP is fixed for each year, and then must be allocated among the states and territories. The initial allocations were based on the number of children and poverty levels, and then changes in subsequent years are based on changes in the number of children in the state. If the number of children declines, however, the state does not have its allocation reduced. This federal funding is then matched by state appropriations. To encourage the expansion of health services to children, the federal government matches state funding at higher rates than it does spending for Medicaid.

Like Medicaid, CHIP is administered by the states, with a significant portion of the funds coming as a matching grant from the federal government. This means of delivering the program has meant that the state governments have had the opportunity to experiment to some extent with the design of the program within their states (Zickafoose, 2020). For example, states may limit the providers to whom CHIP recipients can go for services, and have instituted a version of managed care for the program recipients, in order to save money and coordinate care more effectively.

CHIP does not have the open-ended federal funding that Medicaid does, and therefore may at times impose burdens on state budgets. The administrative costs of CHIP, like other publicly-funded health programs, tend to be significantly lower than for private health insurance programs, but if there are major increases in eligible children, or major increases in the incidence of diseases the states will have to spend more from their own resources. Managed care has helped to control costs in general, but the states still face potential unexpected outlays.

Politics of Medicaid and CHIP

The discussion of federalism, and especially the use of waivers, says a good deal about the elite politics of these two programs, but there are also political questions about the way in which the public regard the programs. Chapter 3 showed that the public tends to have a very positive opinion of Medicare, but public support does not appear to be as strong for Medicaid. This is not a program that most citizens expect to use sometime in their lives, as is true for Medicare. That said, the public do appear to recognize the importance of access to healthcare, including for those citizens who do not have the ability to pay for it.

In a 2019 poll, the Kaiser Family Foundation found that three-quarters of respondents had a favorable view of Medicaid (Table 4.1). As might be expected, Democrats had more favorable views, but even 60 percent of Republican respondents had a favorable view. In an earlier KFF poll (2015) almost 90 percent of respondents said they would enroll themselves or their child in Medicaid if they had no other health insurance. In a 2020 poll, KFF found that more than half of respondents thought that Medicaid worked well (Table 4.2), and in this case more Republicans than Democrats thought it worked well—something that is very unusual for public evaluations of government programs.[4]

Some of the favorable opinion of the public concerning Medicaid is a result of its being seen as a health program rather than a welfare program (Table 4.3). Even though the program is means-tested and goes primarily to the "medically indigent", for a large majority of Americans this is just a health program. There is, perhaps, some halo effect here from Medicare which is clearly a health insurance program without means-testing and which is extremely popular with the public. Indeed, citizens in states that have not expanded Medicaid after passage of the Affordable Care Act now favor the program (see Chapter 5).

Since the initial expansion of Medicaid under the Affordable Care Act there have been seven referendums at the state level concerning expansion. In all but one (Montana) these referendums were successful and Medicaid is being expanded.

Table 4.1: Views of Medicaid (in percentage)

	Very Favorable	Somewhat Favorable	Somewhat Unfavorable	Very Unfavorable
Total	39	36	12	7
Democrats	53	31	8	4
Independents	37	39	12	8
Republicans	27	38	18	9

Source: Kaiser Family Foundation, *Health Tracking Poll*, July 18–20, 2019.

Table 4.2: "Does the current Medicaid program work well for low-income people?" (in percentage)

	Working Well	Not Working Well	Don't Know
Total	56	29	15
Democrats	58	31	12
Independents	55	30	16
Republicans	59	27	14

Source: Kaiser Family Foundation, *Health Tracking Poll*, February 13–18, 2020.

Table 4.3: "Is Medicaid primarily a health insurance or a welfare program?" (in percentage)

	Health	Welfare
Total	67	29
Democrats	78	17
Independents	60	28
Republicans	53	43

Source: Kaiser Family Foundation, *Health Tracking Poll*, February 13–18, 2020.

These referendums have been primarily in deep red states, and appear to show that the public is more supportive of government's role in healthcare than are conservative political elites. Some evidence also indicates that support is especially high among voters with more education and higher incomes, as well as among those who would benefit from the expansion (Matsa and Miller, 2019).

Although there is not as much survey evidence about CHIP, what there is demonstrates that the public considers this a worthwhile program. For example, as shown in Table 4.4, when asked in the early days of the Trump administration about policy priorities, funding CHIP was declared to be the most important action that government should take. This was at a time when defunding CHIP was being floated as a potential means of cutting expenditures, but it was seen as not a viable option by the public. Some proposals widely touted by the Trump administration came farther down the list of policy priorities, including any attempt to repeal the Affordable Care Act.

Perhaps because of the popularity of the programs, the Trump administration, along with Republicans leaders in Congress, attempted to downsize the program, while still claiming to maintain, or even improve, them. This was to be done by converting Medicaid and CHIP into block grant programs, which would permit the states greater latitude in how the money was to be spent. Also, states that accepted the "Healthy Adult Opportunity Medicaid" program would receive lower funding (Mann et al., 2020) but presumably would be focusing on making adults healthier by eliminating some rules. The underlying assumption was, however,

Table 4.4: Priority of CHIP (2017): "Should the following things President Trump and Congress could do in the coming months be a top priority, important but not a top priority, not too important, or should not be done at all?"

	Top Priority	Important but Not Top Priority	Not Too Important	Should Not Be Done
Reauthorizing CHIP Funding	62	26	5	4
Hurricane Relief	61	33	4	2
Stabilizing ACA Marketplace	48	37	7	6
Addressing Prescription Painkiller Epidemic	43	38	12	6
Strengthening Immigration Controls	35	30	18	15
Repealing the ACA	29	22	9	35
Reforming the Tax Code	28	30	13	24

Source: Kaiser Family Foundation, *Health Tracking Poll*, November, 2017.

that, with the fewer rules, the states that wanted to could reduce the number of recipients.

Conclusion

Medicaid and CHIP emphasize the "jungle" nature of healthcare in the United States. Medicaid is a nominally federal program, but the manner in which the program is administered through the states makes access to healthcare something of a lottery for citizens. Depending on where they live, they will receive different levels of service, and may or may not be eligible for Medicaid at all. This inequality in access appears to be becoming even more evident, as "red" states attempt to make access more difficult. The courts have protected citizens somewhat from the worst political ploys to remove access, as has legislation preserving coverage during the pandemic, but there is still a gradual degradation of the program in many states.

The jungle aspect of the program can also be seen in the administrative burdens placed on any applicants for the program. The majority of the effort required to gain eligibility for Medicaid must be done by citizens (Herd et al., 2013). This administrative choice is apparently done to save the states money in personnel, and also to limit uptake of the program in some states. This places the burden of fighting through a jungle of paperwork on citizens who tend to be less educated than average and who may not be familiar with all the terms within the application.

The administrative burdens of Medicaid and CHIP do not, however, fall entirely on the citizens, and the states must confront a jungle of their own. These administrative demands are especially evident if they want to make changes from the basic guidelines of the program through the waiver process. Many states have wanted to do things such as add work requirements to the program, and that has involved major investments of time and energy. The waiver process also emphasizes the political nature of this program (and others) given that some types of waivers are easier to obtain than are others, depending upon which party controls the executive branch of government.

5

Affordable Care Act: a major step forward

The most significant piece of health policy legislation in American history was signed into law on March 23, 2010 by President Barack Obama. The Patient Protection and Affordable Care Act, usually referred to as the Affordable Care Act (ACA), or simply "Obamacare", is an attempt to make health insurance available to all Americans. This legislation has made more affordable health insurance available to anyone who wishes to purchase it and, although it is far from a panacea for all the problems within the healthcare system, it has increased access significantly. The ACA's principal provisions came into effect in 2014, and by 2018 the number of uninsured in the United States was roughly halved (CBO, 2020).

The passage of the ACA was the culmination of a long struggle for some form of national healthcare coverage that began with President Theodore Roosevelt, a Republican, around the beginning of the twentieth century. Several Democratic presidents after that time—Franklin Roosevelt, Harry Truman and Bill Clinton—had made efforts of varying intensity to adopt a program of this sort, but had all failed. They had encountered the general American skepticism about "socialized medicine", as well as the political power of groups such as the American Medical Association and the health insurance industry.

Although it has been a success in many ways (see below) the ACA has been a major source of political contention since its passage. Indeed, getting the legislation through Congress was far from easy, and relied upon the relatively uncommon occurrence of both houses of Congress and the presidency controlled by the same party.[1] Even then, although the legislation had passed under the regular rules of the Senate, a set of crucial amendments had to be passed under the special rules of reconciliation that prevent a filibuster (DeBonis, 2016). Republicans in Congress have mounted dozens of attempts to repeal the Act, even while Obama was in office. One did pass Congress but was promptly vetoed by President Obama. Even when Donald Trump was president, and would certainly have approved of the repeal, the Republicans in Congress were unsuccessful.[2] As Jonathan Cohn (2021, 325) wrote "There was plenty that Americans did not like about the Affordable Care Act. But they did not want to go back".

Although the ACA was a major political and policy accomplishment, and has made major contributions to improving access to healthcare, it is far from a perfect piece of legislation. As I will develop in this chapter, the Act is complex, depends perhaps too much on private insurers, and had one major provision that proved to be unconstitutional. Even with the success of the ACA, millions of Americans do not have health insurance, and many millions more do not have the full coverage envisioned by the framers of the legislation but depend on high deductible policies. Obamacare has been a first step toward improving access, but there is a great deal that remains to be done.

Background of the Affordable Care Act

Improving healthcare was a major issue in the 2008 presidential elections, especially in the Democratic primaries. During the primary campaign Barack Obama advocated a healthcare insurance plan that would be provided by the public sector, somewhat similar to what is now known as "Medicare for All". His principal opponent in the primaries, Hillary Clinton, proposed a plan more like the final ACA legislation. Her plan would depend upon an individual mandate—all citizens would be required to have health insurance, whether provided by employers, by government, or purchased individually from private insurance companies.

The plan proposed by Hillary Clinton during the primaries was essentially the plan developed by Senator Lincoln Chafee (R-RI) as the Republican response to the proposal by the (Bill) Clinton administration in 1993. The Clinton administration had proposed a plan that depended on subsidized health insurance for all citizens, paid for by employers and government (Enthoven, 1994). This program would have been a replacement for Medicaid, as well as for conventional employer-provided health insurance. Because it relied on private insurers, Senator Chafee's plan was more acceptable to conservative Republicans, and indeed was advocated by the extremely conservative Heritage Foundation. In addition, the Chafee plan had been adopted in Massachusetts when Mitt Romney, a Republican and later (2012) a presidential candidate against Obama, was governor.

The Clinton plan failed rather dramatically (Donnelly and Rochefort, 2012), and Obama's plan in the primaries was somewhat reminiscent of its emphasis on providing insurance through the public sector. However, once elected, President Obama was faced with a Congress that was not yet ready for such a sweeping plan that could have undermined private health insurance—one of the most powerful industries, and one of the most powerful lobbies, in Washington. Thus, although he was inaugurated in January, 2009 the healthcare legislation was not adopted until March, 2010 (see Cahn and Johnston, 2018), and during that year President Obama largely allowed Congress to design the legislation. The "Gang of Six"— three Democrats and three Republicans—was especially important in designing the legislation and then getting it passed (Frates and Brown, 2009).

The bill that was adopted was more similar to Hillary Clinton's, and Mitt Romney's, plan than that which Obama had discussed in his campaign.[3] The program depended upon an individual mandate to be insured, and the ability to purchase health insurance from private sector providers. Given its historical links with the Republican party, there was initial support from Republicans, but that changed significantly as the Bill came closer to passage. There were numerous claims that the mandate was unconstitutional and that the legislation would undermine employer-provided health insurance, which was popular with those employees who had it. In the end, the legislation in its final form, with crucial amendments, could only be passed in the Senate through the reconciliation process.[4]

Principal provisions of the Affordable Care Act

The ACA is an extensive and complex piece of legislation over 1,000 pages in length. While the major purpose of the legislation was to make health insurance accessible to all Americans the legislation affected almost all aspects of healthcare. The legislation was focused on access, but also had major provisions that dealt with cost and the quality of care. Some of the components of the legislation were to be phased in over a period of up to a decade. Beginning with access policies, I will now present some of the major provisions of the program, and discuss their strengths and weaknesses.

Individual mandate

As already discussed, the individual mandate to have health insurance was a central feature of the ACA. Further, not only did individuals have to have insurance; initially, the insurance they purchased or received as a benefit of employment had to cover a range of possible diseases and treatments,[5] and would have to have some emphasis on preventative care. The emphasis on prevention was not only to improve the health of the insured; it was designed to save the program money in the long run.

If individuals did not have health insurance they would have to pay a penalty. That penalty was to be paid along with the income tax, and was based on income levels or a flat amount per person in the household, whichever was greater (see Table 5.1). The idea behind the mandate was not only to try to have as complete coverage as possible, but also to guard against a possible "death spiral" that would occur without it. Without the mandate, healthier, younger people might not buy insurance, thus making the costs of the insurance higher for a pool that is more likely to need medical interventions. As rates rose in response to greater use of medical care, more people would be willing to take the risk and would drop out, raising rates even higher. For the insurance to be affordable, the pool of participants must be as broad as possible.

President Obama was initially opposed to the individual mandate, but accepted it once the potential threats to the program were made clear. This provision continued to be, however, one of the major points of political contention around the ACA. Republicans, and a few Democrats, argued that government should not be in the business of making people buy a particular product, comparing buying health insurance to buying broccoli. This argument ignored the fact that state governments had for many years required automobile owners to buy insurance, and the mandate was approved by the Supreme Court (see p. 75).

The individual mandate was repealed, effective in 2019, by the Trump administration in the Tax Cuts and Jobs Act of 2017 (Jost, 2017). There was

Table 5.1: Original penalty for not being insured

The penalty was calculated as the greater of either:

1) a percentage of the "applicable income", defined as the amount by which an individual's household income exceeds the applicable filing threshold for the applicable tax year. The filing threshold comprises the personal exemption amount (doubled for those married filing jointly) plus the standard deduction amount.

  • the percentage would be 1.0% in 2014, 2.0% in 2015, and 2.5% thereafter

2) a flat dollar amount assessed on each taxpayer and any dependents (for example, family)

  • the annual flat dollar amount phased in—$95 in 2014, $325 in 2015, and $695 in 2016 and beyond (adjusted for inflation), assessed for each taxpayer and any dependents,

  • the amount was reduced by one-half for dependents under the age of 18,
  • the total family penalty was capped at 300% of the annual flat dollar amount.

However, the penalty for noncompliance cannot exceed the national average premium for Bronze-level-qualified health plans offered through exchanges (for the relevant family size).

Source: Chaikind (2010).

no longer a federal individual mandate, although five states and the District of Columbia have retained some form of mandate. It was hoped by Republicans that eliminating the mandate would effectively kill Obamacare entirely, but this was not the case. By 2019 enough people had become accustomed to having health insurance through the ACA that they did not want to give it up. Further, the beginning of the COVID-19 pandemic shortly after the repeal of the mandate helped emphasize the importance of having health insurance.

In addition to the individual mandate, the ACA contained a mandate for employers with over 50 full-time employees to provide health insurance for the employees. Critics of this provision argued that it created a perverse incentive to convert full-time employees to part-time (Kliff, 2013). There was indeed some increase in the amount of part-time employment, with some companies topping out employment at 29 hours (30 hours defined full time), but the effect seems to have been minor. There were also criticisms that this provision would slow the growth of smaller companies (the 50th employee would become extremely expensive).

Exchanges and insurance

Under the ACA individuals were to purchase their health insurance through "exchanges" in each state. These exchanges are websites that list the available policies in the state, and allow the individual to purchase one of a number of plans. Likewise, insurance companies would make their plans available on these exchanges. There are four types of plans available through the exchanges—Bronze, Silver,

Gold and Platinum. They have the same coverages of conditions and services, but differ in the size of the premium and the sizes of the deductibles. Bronze plans, for example, have low monthly premiums but have higher deductibles before the plan begins to pay[6] while Platinum plans have higher premiums but lower deductibles and co-pays. A younger individual, for example, who did not think that he or she would need to use the insurance much, might opt for higher deductibles, and therefore might save some money.

The insurance available through the exchanges is subsidized by the federal government through the income tax system. This subsidy comes in two forms. The first is that there is a maximum premium that the insured must pay, based on their income relative to the federal poverty line (see Table 5.2). In addition, there is a maximum out-of-pocket payment for the insured, also based on levels of income. These subsidies are intended to make insurance affordable; but still for many people health insurance could consume close to 10 percent of their income. In addition to the subsidy that comes in the amount of the premium paid, there is a maximum amount that individuals must pay out of pocket as a percentage of their income. Those at or below 133 percent of the poverty level (this lower number depends upon the state: see Chapter 4) are enrolled in Medicaid, but those between 133 percent and 200 percent pay 3 percent of income, and those between 200 and 300 percent pay a maximum 6.3 percent. Those above 300 percent of the poverty level ($83,250 in 2022 for a family of four) can pay up to 9.3 percent. While this subsidized insurance is more affordable than insurance on the unsubsidized market, it still constitutes a major share of many people's income. In addition to the subsidized plans for individuals, there are some small subsidies available for small businesses who offer insurance to their employees.

While the policies offered by the ACA are subsidized, the subsidies were increased during the COVID-19 pandemic. The American Rescue Plan adopted in March, 2021 expanded the subsidy for people above 400 percent of the poverty line, and reduced the premiums for most insured. This additional subsidy was available for 2021 and 2022, and the Biden administration attempted to extend it as part of its "Build Back Better" plan, but that plan has not been passed and.

Table 5.2: Maximum net premiums after subsidies for a family of four (2019)

Income % of federal poverty level	Premium cap as share of income	Maximum annual net premium after subsidy	Maximum out-of-pocket
133	3.11% of income	$1,038	$5,200
150	4.15% of income	$1,562	$5,200
200	6.54% of income	$3,283	$5,200
250	8.36% of income	$5,246	$12,600
300	9.86% of income	$7,425	$15,800
400	9.86% of income	$9,899	$15,800

Note: The numbers in the table do not apply for Alaska and Hawaii.
Source: Healthcare.gov, https://www.healthcare.gov/glossary/out-of-pocket-maximum-limit/.

many people began to pay much higher premiums as of January 1, 2023 (Cox et al., 2022).

The insurance offered under the ACA covers a full range of conditions and treatments. The insurance has a greater emphasis on prevention than does most private health insurance, and preventative care is provided without co-payments or deductibles. The program is also oriented toward children's health, providing a full range of coverage, including dental (not available for adults). The ACA plans were also to cover contraception, but later court rulings enabled some small businesses not to offer this coverage (see p. 75). Given the state-based nature of health insurance markets, each state could define the details of the "essential health benefits" offered in the plans in their state, within the guidelines established by the program.

Under the ACA individuals can still use high-deductible health plans and health savings accounts (HSAs), and some of these are offered on the exchanges. These policies have lower costs than the more complete plans, but still must offer services such as preventative care. Also, under the ACA there is a maximum allowable out-of-pocket expenditure ($7,000 for individuals and $14,000 for families). With the high deductible plan individuals using an HSA can receive tax breaks for contributing to the plan, and then have access to the money when needed for medical expenditures (Robinson, 2005).

One of the crucial elements of the plans offered under the ACA was that no one could be denied coverage because of pre-existing conditions. This provision was important to ensure access to health insurance for patients who might ordinarily be rejected in the private market. This provision was also important for economic reasons because people who had chronic conditions, or who had had major diseases in the past, might be locked into an employer and the insurance they already had, thus limiting labor mobility. Further, the requirement to insure potentially very expensive individuals made the individual mandate all the more important for maintaining the solvency of these plans. Although potentially expensive, the coverage of pre-existing conditions is one of the aspects of the ACA most popular with the public.

The original plan for the exchanges was for there to be a separate exchange for each state, in part because insurance markets are still primarily organized on a state-by-state basis. If a state could not, or would not, create its own exchange then the federal government would have an exchange that would serve the citizens of that state. As of March 2023, 21 states and the District of Columbia have their own exchanges and the other states use the federal exchange.[7] Not surprisingly the states with their own exchanges tend to be "blue", with more liberal politics and greater initial support for the ACA (see Haeder and Weimer, 2013).

Launching the exchanges was something of a debacle (Sanger-Katz and Kliff, 2021). While many of the state exchanges performed as planned, the federal exchange, which was to handle a large share of the business, was slow to start and often crashed. This failure was perhaps because of the volume of business, and perhaps because the designer had little experience with designing websites for services of this sort. For whatever reason, the slow and erratic start of the exchange was seen by many as an indication of the likely overall failure of the program.

Medicaid expansion

The discussion of insurance plans offered under the ACA has a base of 133 percent of the poverty line. The ACA mandated that the states expand Medicaid to insure people at this level of income or below, which would have involved an expansion of coverage by Medicaid in a number of states (especially in the South and West). This expansion was important for the success of the program in making healthcare become more universal. Individuals and families at or below that level of income would face great difficulties in paying even for subsidized health insurance. The states were given an incentive to make this expansion—all the costs of expanding Medicaid would be paid by the federal government for the first ten years, and most of it would be covered in the following years.

This financial incentive might appear to be too good an opportunity for the states to ignore. They could improve health insurance access to their citizens at no cost. Despite that incentive, a number of states did choose not to expand Medicaid, and sued in federal court saying that the mandate on the states was an unconstitutional expansion of federal power within a federal system. The states won that suit (Rosenbaum and Westmoreland, 2012) when the court ruled that the federal government lacked the authority to make states spend money in certain ways. As a result, some ten states have not yet expanded coverage. As discussed in Chapter 4 on Medicaid, however, several states, including some with the most conservative politics in the country, have been forced by popular referendums to expand coverage.

Cost containment

Given that the federal government was now taking a more central position in healthcare, it became even more interested in controlling costs. The ACA contained a number of provisions directed toward cost control and efficiency. One of the simplest was a mandate that the insurers spend at least 80 percent of premiums (increasing over time to 85 percent) on care. This prevented excessive profits on the part of the insurance companies, and required any insurer that did not spend that much to give rebates to its clients. For example, in 2022 insurers had to issue over $1 billion in rebates to the insured (Ortaliza et al., 2022)

The ACA also provided support for accountable care organizations (ACOs). These organizations are analogous to health maintenance organizations in that the members pay an annual fee for all their medical care. ACOs are typically organized by doctors or hospitals, and they have not been very successful. This lack of success has been in large part the result of underestimating the risks involved with creating organizations when they may include some patients who had not had good health insurance previously, and would therefore require more treatments to get in good health.

Taxation

The ACA involved spending a good deal of additional federal money on healthcare, in addition to the significant amounts that were already being spent for Medicare, Medicaid, CHIP (the Children's Health Insurance Program) and a host of other programs. The legislation therefore contained several new taxes that would to some extent offset the expenditures. These taxes were directed primarily at more affluent Americans, and those who already had good healthcare coverage through their employers or from purchasing individual policies in the market.

The major source of new revenue was an expansion of the Medicare tax that was already being collected. Prior to the adoption of the ACA this was a payroll tax of 1.45 percent of income for all employers and all employees.[8] After the passage of the Act income over $200,000 for individuals ($250,000 for couples) was taxed at an additional rate of 0.9 percent. In addition to the payroll tax there is a so-called "Cadillac" tax on very expensive employer-provided health insurance plans, but the implementation of that tax continues to be delayed. There were also several minor excise taxes, including one on tanning salons[9] that have since been repealed.

Consequences of the Affordable Care Act

The major goal of the ACA was to increase access to medical care for Americans, and there was a substantial extension of health insurance coverage because of the Act. As shown in Table 5.3, millions of people have signed up for health insurance through the Act, although the numbers with insurance have varied somewhat over time. There was an initial surge of people signing up for the new opportunity for coverage, and there has been a second surge of enrollment during the COVID-19 pandemic. It appears that Obamacare is now institutionalized as a means through which a significant number of citizens can receive insurance.

All the additions of coverage do not, of course, come through signing up for policies through the exchanges. For example, in 2016, the Congressional Budget Office analyzed the results of the ACA (see Table 5.3) and found that 24 million

Table 5.3: Increased insurance coverage resulting from the Affordable Care Act, 2016 (in millions)

Medicaid Expansion	Subsidized Insurance	Unsubsidized Insurance	Other	Total
11	10	2	1	24

Source: CBO (2016).

people had received coverage because of Obamacare (CBO, 2016). Of those, 11 million received coverage because of the Medicaid expansion, while slightly fewer received coverage because of insurance through the exchanges with a subsidy, and two million got coverage without the subsidy. Approximately one million received other forms of coverage, such as some changes in Medicare coverage.

Problems with the Affordable Care Act

While the ACA has made major contributions to improving the health of Americans, it is far from a panacea for all the problems that exist within the healthcare system. Some of the problems, such as the reliance on private firms, are endemic in American healthcare, but some have been created by the way in which the legislation has been written. These problems within the ACA have led to demands for repeal by some critics, and demands for continued reform, and for moving toward a system that is more publicly funded, by others.

Politically, these problems demonstrate the importance of feedback, and the political effects of policy adoption. The initial passage of the ACA was to a great extent a partisan and ideological battle between right and left. Once the legislation was adopted, however, the nature of the politics has become more technical, and it has become more about the specific effects of the legislation, and the need to amend or repeal it (see Oberlander and Weaver, 2015). The legislation has created some new coalitions and new reasons for support or opposition of the program, and hence a second and subsequent rounds of politics have been evolving.

Subsidy cliff

The ACA builds in a version of the "poverty trap" (Barrett and McPeak, 2006), in which a small increase in income can mean a major loss of subsidies—in the case of the ACA meaning a major increase in premiums. The cut-off of subsidies at higher income levels, both before the extra subsidies during the pandemic and after that subsidy was introduced, could produce major losses for insured families. Earning a few additional dollars could mean paying several hundred dollars extra a month in premiums and out-of-pocket payments. While the insured may not always make those calculations when they have the opportunity to earn more money, it could be a significant disincentive to individual economic advancement.

Family glitch

The ACA provides healthcare subsidies for policies if those do exceed 9.5 percent of income. If, however, an individual policy provided by an employer for the employee meets that standard then the individual and his or her family cannot receive tax credits for purchasing a policy. The difficulty is that the *family* policy offered by the employer may be more than the 9.5 percent threshold while the individual policy is not, so the family is faced with the option of paying very high costs or doing without insurance. It is estimated that this "glitch" affects five million people in 2022, over half children (Jost, 2022).

The Biden administration proposed a change to the rules used by the Internal Revenue Service (IRS) to implement the tax subsidy provision of the ACA.[10] This change in the regulations was adopted in time for the 2023 open enrollment period for the ACA. The new rule requires the IRS to consider not only the cost of the individual policy offered by the employer but also the expenses that would be incurred if a family policy were purchased. The employer plan must now meet a "minimum value" test of covering at least 60 percent of total allowed costs for the entire family, not just the worker (Keith, 2022).

Reliance on the states

Healthcare has historically been a major state activity, and federal programs existing at the time of the adoption of the ACA, notably Medicaid, also relied heavily on the states. Two of the major provisions of the ACA—the expansion of Medicaid and the development of state exchanges—depended on the states, and in some cases the state governments were unwilling to rise to the challenge. Much of the failure of the states had to do with partisan politics, which is a common problem in implementing programs within a federal structure (Adam et al., 2019). Republican-led governments in states in the South and Midwest were simply unwilling to cooperate with a program that they considered to be "socialized medicine".[11] President Biden's fiscal year 2024 budget did, however, contain provisions to provide Medicaid-like coverage even in those states (Park, 2023).

Complexity

One of the principal problems with the ACA is that the legislation and its implementation is so complex. This legislation has created its own jungle within the larger jungle of American healthcare. Implementing the Act involves hundreds of actors, including the 50 state governments, and attempting to deliver health policy coherently is extremely challenging (Bêland et al., 2019). Many people enrolling in the program have expressed frustration with the difficulties of deciding among plans, and with making the exchange websites function properly. Of course, those individuals who lack their own access to the internet encounter even greater difficulties.

The ACA has affected not only individual citizens but the healthcare industry as well. Doctors and hospitals have been confronted with a new set of regulations to follow and a host of new patients to serve. While most medical practitioners do laud the increases in access, and the emphasis on preventative care, they are far from enamored with the increased regulations and "red tape" (Scott, 2017). The complexity of the legislation reflects in part the difficulties in building a coalition to pass the legislation and the need to satisfy a range of political constituencies in a single piece of legislation.

Loss of insurers

The idea of the exchanges was that citizens would have choices, not only among the levels of coverage in the plan (Bronze, Silver, Gold and Platinum) but also among various insurance providers for each type of plan. That goal has proven more difficult to reach than initially thought, given that the insurers found it difficult to estimate risks before the plans were actually operating, and therefore it was difficult to set premiums that would allow them to make a profit (Griffith et al., 2018). Later, insurers in some states found that the risk pools were too small to enable them to continue offering the plans with a reasonable level of risk and dropped out of the exchanges.

These problems with keeping insurers involved has meant that one state—Delaware—has only one option available in its exchanges. This is a state with a small population and hence a small risk pool. Further, given that there are different insurance regulators in each state, complying with different regulations for a small market may not be worthwhile. Further, given that insurers may operate in some counties and not others within a state, some counties in 15 other states have only one provider (McDermott and Cox, 2020).[12] Some of the larger states, for example California and New York, have six to ten more insurers offering plans. This disparity in the availability of competitive insurance providers is another example of the difficulties posed by depending upon state-level organizations, with differing regulations, to manage the insurance.

Costs

Finally, the costs of the insurance offered to individuals, and the tendency for the costs to increase, has disappointed and angered some enrollees in the program. It is important to remember that many of the people enrolled in health insurance through the ACA may not have had health insurance previously and are not accustomed to the charges. Further, many are among the "working poor" who have limited resources and find the health insurance fees a significant addition to their regular expenses.

This cost factor has been one of the important factors driving political reactions among the public, especially the members of the public who might be thought to support the ACA. For example, in one county in Kentucky the rate of uninsured dropped by 60 percent, but 82 percent of the voters voted for Donald Trump in 2016 (Kliff, 2016). Many of these voters wanted something done about the costs of the program, and thought Trump would help them. Despite an attempt to repeal the program, and the elimination of the personal mandate, the Trump administration did little to change the ACA (Oberlander, 2018).

Myths about Obamacare

There are some genuine problems with Obamacare, but the political conflicts over the program also produced a number of mythical problems that have been developed largely for political reasons. Despite the absence of any factual foundation, these assumed "problems" in the program were powerful politically, and appeared again and again in the debates over the Act. Even years into the implementation of the ACA, the same myths continue to be repeated in opposition to the program.

Death panels

Sarah Palin, former governor of Alaska and the Republican vice-presidential candidate in 2008, claimed in 2009 that Obamacare would create "death panels" composed of bureaucrats who would decide who was worthy of care under the program, and who would be allowed to die. This claim arose from a provision in the original legislation that paid physicians to counsel patients, especially elderly patients, about living wills and other end-of-life decisions (Davis, 2009). Palin's false claim created so much controversy during debates on the legislation that the provision was deleted from the final legislation.

The death panel myth has been perpetuated in part by the Independent Payment Advisory Board created by the ACA. This body was designed to advise the Department of Health and Human Services about possible cost-saving possibilities in Medicare, including evaluating the cost-effectiveness of certain types of treatment (Ebeler et al., 2011). The body was forbidden from making any such recommendations before 2020, and even then would certainly not be advising about individual patient treatment. That reality of the board did not prevent the spreading of another version of the death panel rumor.

Coverage

Several myths about coverages available under the ACA arose, and continue to appear. The first was that Congress itself did not like the coverage and would have their own insurance plan. This pattern of coverage was in fact true *before* the passage of the ACA, but the legislation required members of Congress and their staffs to obtain their insurance through the exchanges or through some other government-provided plan, for example Medicare. There was also a myth that coverage under the ACA was available to illegal immigrants, but this was not true.

President Obama himself was responsible for one of the more important myths concerning coverage under the plan. Numerous times during the campaign for the Bill Obama said that "if you like your plan, you can keep it", meaning that people with health insurance would not be forced to get new insurance. However, in 2013 millions of people received notices that their existing policies were canceled. As noted above, the ACA created standards that all health insurance policies had to meet in order to fulfill the individual mandate, and those that did not were canceled. These cancellations produced a major embarrassment for the president, and the administration had to apologize, while also arguing that the plans individuals would then have to buy would provide more benefits than those that had been voided.

Affordable Care Act and the Supreme Court

Any complicated and intrusive piece of legislation such as the ACA is likely, within the American litigious political system (Kagan, 2003), to produce a number of suits about its constitutionality. This was certainly true of the ACA. Many of the major provisions of the Act have been litigated, and there have been wins and losses for both the federal government and the opponents of the Act. But, despite some losses, the basics of the ACA remain in place and are becoming more institutionalized.

The first, and potentially most damaging, suit challenged the individual mandate as exceeding the powers of the federal government. The Supreme Court ruled, however, in *National Federation of Independent Business v Sibelius*[13] that the mandate and the requirement to purchase insurance or pay a penalty was in reality a tax and was therefore well within the powers of the federal government.[14] The same case, however, invalidated the provision of the Act mandating that the states expand Medicaid eligibility or lose their Medicaid funding. This was deemed to be excessive coercion of the state governments. In a later decision, *King v Burwell*,[15] the court ruled that even though the legislation was written in terms of each state having its own exchanges, the subsidies in the Act could still be paid in states that used the federal exchange.

The next major challenge was over the requirement in the law that insurance policies provide for contraception. In several court cases, notably *Little Sisters of the Poor Saints Peter and Paul Home v Pennsylvania*[16] and *Burwell v Hobby Lobby Stores*[17] the Supreme Court ruled that an employer that disapproved for reasons of religion or conscience of the requirement for contraception in policies offered through the ACA did not have to provide that coverage. This ruling, of course, left many women working for these organizations to fend for themselves to receive any birth control services they may have wanted.

Finally, in *California v Texas*[18] the court upheld a challenge to the constitutionality of the entire Act after the Tax Cut and Jobs Act of 2017 had eliminated the "tax" created by the individual mandate. The state of Texas sued, saying the Act was therefore illegal since it was not related to any specific powers granted Congress. The US Department of Justice in the Trump administration would not defend the Act, but the state of California and several other states did defend it. After going through several moves up and down within the federal court system, the Supreme Court ruled that Texas did not have standing to sue,[19] and therefore the Act could remain in effect.

Given the ideological shift of the Supreme Court during the Trump administration, there may well be additional legal challenges to the ACA. Although the public has now widely accepted the Act and the principle of greater public involvement in healthcare, many elites in the Republican party at the state level have not. They may attempt to find means to bring new cases to the Supreme Court and overturn the program, despite the inability of political challenges to do so.

Public opinion and the Affordable Care Act

As already mentioned, the ACA has been one of the major points of contention between the parties, and among citizens, since the discussion about it began in 2009. This controversy if anything intensified after the passage of the legislation, as politicians and citizens began to understand what the legislation would actually do to healthcare in the United States. Some of that discussion was based on myths and poor understandings of health policy, but much of it reflected genuine ideological differences, as well as different commitments to the principle that healthcare was a fundamental right of citizenship.

At the time of the passage of the ACA only about a third of the public supported the program, with a large number of people being uncertain about it. Some of the opposition was a dislike of anything that looked like "socialized medicine", while others feared that it would undermine either their own health insurance plans, or Medicare, or both. Still others thought that there would be too many new patients brought into the healthcare system, and that the quality of care for all patients would suffer. Although opposition continues, panel research has shown that the intensity of opposition to the ACA has been declining (Jacobs et al., 2019).

The supporters of the ACA, on the other hand, have generally favored the extension of adequate health insurance to more of the population, and many have been themselves beneficiaries of the program (Jacobs et al., 2019). Many supporters would have preferred a more public bill, but have been willing to accept that the perfect is often the enemy of the good, and understand that this legislation has made a significant difference in the lives of many Americans. Somewhat surprisingly, labor unions were not strong advocates of the ACA both because their members often had good insurance through their employers that might be put in jeopardy, and because some activists favored a more public option (Fraser, 2013).

Table 5.4 shows the changes in public opinion concerning the ACA from just before its passage through to 2022. In the period before the actual implementation of the Act public opinion tended to be negative, and this encouraged many of the Republican attempts at repeal. However, after the Act began to be implemented in 2014 the favorable opinions among the public tended to increase, and there is now a solid majority in favor of the program. As already noted, the American public has become accustomed to having more access to health insurance as well as having additional protections, such as coverage for pre-existing conditions and coverage of adult children who are still students.

As might be expected, there are marked differences among respondents based on their political affiliations, with Democrats being much more favorable to the ACA and Republicans being very opposed (Table 5.4). Independents initially were much closer to Republicans in their view, with fewer than one-third

Table 5.4: Public opinion on the Affordable Care Act (percent favorable; last survey each year)

	Total	Democrat	Independent	Republican
2010	42	68	37	15
2011	43	64	33	19
2012	43	72	37	14
2013	34	68	28	7
2014	41	69	40	10
2015	40	67	32	14
2016	43	70	42	18
2017	50	80	43	17
2018	53	81	46	17
2019	53	82	53	22
2020	53	80	55	19
2021	58	85	55	28
2022	55	87	58	21

Source: Kaiser Family Foundation, *Health Tracking Poll*, Monthly.

Table 5.5: Age and opinion on the Affordable Care Act (January, 2022)

	Favorable	Unfavorable
18–29	56	38
30–49	65	35
50–64	53	42
65+	50	41

Source: Kaiser Family Foundation, *Health Tracking Poll*, March, 2022.

supporting Obamacare, but over time they have become more positive. Indeed, over time Republicans have become more favorable although still over half oppose the legislation.

Other factors such as age also influence levels of support for the ACA (Table 5.5). For example, although all age groups tended to be more favorable than unfavorable toward the ACA, those respondents aged 30–49 were the most supportive. These individuals find the Act has helped them with supporting their families. Those 65 and older were the least supportive, perhaps because they already had Medicare and hence saw no personal benefit. Younger respondents also supported the legislation. This group has tended to be more progressive and to favor some form of national health insurance. This is true even though many younger people have chosen to take their chances without buying Obamacare insurance after the mandate ended. These younger voters also tend to favor replacement of the ACA with a more comprehensive, single-payer plan for healthcare.

Repeal of the Affordable Care Act

The information on public opinion makes it clear that Republicans are not supportive of the ACA and almost since its adoption there have been attempts to repeal the legislation. By 2014 when the Act was implemented there had been 54 attempts to repeal the ACA (O'Keefe, 2014) in the House of Representatives. By 2017, the number had risen to 70. To some extent these efforts before 2017 were symbolic, given that it was clear that President Obama would veto repeal and there would not be a sufficient majority to override the veto. By 2017 the threat to the legislation was more real, given that President Trump would have gladly signed the repeal legislation.

At the beginning, these efforts at repeal were useful to Republicans in Congress because their voters tended not to support the ACA, but over time, as the Act has become more popular, the political calculus has changed somewhat. Now even a significant number of Republican voters support Obamacare. One major problem that the Republicans in Congress have had with their attempts to repeal is that they have not had a clear and plausible alternative to Obamacare. The political rhetoric was in terms of "repeal and replace", but there was rarely a well-developed plan for replacement. There was some advocacy of HSAs, and other mechanisms that put the burden on the individual (Robinson, 2005), but no options that would be able to address the needs of the millions of citizens who had received health insurance because of the ACA.

Conclusion

The ACA represents a major political achievement for President Obama, and a major advance in health policy in the United States. For the first time there were publicly supported insurance policies available to anyone, regardless of age or income. These policies filled in a major gap in coverage, and brought millions more Americans under an insurance umbrella as they confronted the high costs of medical care. The legislation also added a number of regulations that helped to stabilize costs and improve quality, even in the face of significantly increased access that might have driven costs much higher, and quality lower.

At the same time, the ACA represents something of a failure. President Obama and many of his supporters had wanted a more public version, with the insurance being provided by government rather than by private insurers. This might also have eliminated the need for the involvement of state governments through eliminating Medicaid. Millions of people were added to the ranks of the insured, but millions also continued to be uninsured or underinsured, and the complexity of the program adds many administrative challenges. This was a major step on the route to a more comprehensive approach to healthcare access in the United States, but it will almost certainly not be the final step along that path.

6

Regulatory policies in healthcare

Most of the discussion about health policy in the United States is about access, and the insurance programs that attempt to ensure that people have access to medical care. These programs are certainly important for individual participants, and taken together play a major role in shaping national health outcomes. But these programs are not the only way in which government intervenes in healthcare, and the regulatory programs managed by all levels of government are important for the quality, and the costs, of healthcare, as well as affecting public health outcomes. These programs rely primarily on law, rather than money, to produce changes in the provision of health. Regulation is one of the principal instruments available to government to achieve its policy goals (Pancheco-Vega, 2020) and often is a lower cost and less intrusive form of public sector intervention than the provision of insurance.

This chapter will focus on health regulation at the federal level, but it is important to remember that a great deal of regulatory activity is undertaken by the states and by local governments. For example, states license physicians, nurses and other health professionals. They also inspect healthcare facilities such as hospitals and nursing homes. They are also involved in environmental health, such as controls over air and water pollution. Local governments regulate a number of areas that are important for health, such as the cleanliness of food stores and restaurants. They also provide water and sanitation services and, when those are unavailable, regulate the private alternatives. Local governments are also involved in regulating environmental causes of disease, and in controlling highly transmissible diseases.

Although discussed more often in terms of access and quality, there is also a major regulatory role for programs such as Medicare and the Affordable Care Act. For example, Medicare regulates the facilities that its recipients utilize, such as hospitals, hospices and nursing homes, as well as general regulations on the quality of care provided to its recipients. The Affordable Care Act imposed more controls over the practice of medicine, including requirements for greater screening and preventative care and an emphasis on patient satisfaction.

Regulation of pharmaceuticals

The major area of federal regulation in healthcare is the approval of pharmaceuticals and medical appliances. At the beginning of the twentieth century there were virtually no restrictions on what could be sold as a medicine, nor were there restrictions on the advertising claims that could be made about those "medicines" (Young, 1961). The same lack of regulation afflicted the food industry, with little or no guarantees of the purity of food being sold. It is impossible to make a definitive statement about the consequences of this unregulated market, but certainly it cost the lives of thousands, if not millions, of citizens.

The open wide market in medicines began to change with the Pure Food and Drug Act passed by Congress in 1906. This Act was placed on the agenda of government in part by the "muckraking" journalism and literature of the time that exposed the dangers of the lack of regulation. Perhaps the most famous book in this literature is *The Jungle*, by Upton Sinclair (1906; see also Sarin and Sarin, 2002).[1] While Sinclair's book focused on food, specifically meat packing, it helped to shine light more generally on the range of dangers existing in the market at that time.[2]

Although the Pure Food and Drug Act, and the creation of the Food and Drug Administration (FDA) through the Act, marks the real beginning of drug regulation in the United States, it is important to note that during the administration of Abraham Lincoln the Bureau of Chemistry was created in the Department of Agriculture. It undertook some analyses of possible adulterants in food, and to a very minor extent drugs. However, given that it was in the Department of Agriculture—dedicated to serving the interests of farmers and the rest of the food industry—there was a very strong possibility of regulatory capture. Therefore, it was important to create a review process of food and medicines that was more autonomous.

The Pure Food and Drug Act was a legislative milestone, but it did not establish a very strong process for dealing with food and pharmaceuticals. The major emphasis was on the purity of food and drugs, and the elimination of substances that could be harmful to consumers. The Act also required labeling of all the ingredients of a medicine, although those standards were not nearly as stringent as contemporary standards. Further, there was as yet no authority to assess the efficacy of drugs— as long as they contained no adulterants that was all that was legally required to market the food or medicine.

The powers of the FDA were expanded under the Food, Drug and Cosmetics Act of 1938. As the name implies, this Act gave the FDA the authority to regulate cosmetics in addition to its ongoing responsibilities.[3] The Act also enabled the FDA to assess the safety of the ingredients in drugs, not just to exclude dangerous substances that might be adulterating the medicine. The FDA could prevent a medicine being sold if it found the ingredients to be unsafe or mislabeled. The FDA was also given the power to inspect where drugs were being manufactured, and to assess the cleanliness of those premises and the possibilities of contamination. There was not, however, any legal difference yet between prescription and non-prescription drugs (until 1951) so that many substances now tightly regulated were easily obtainable.

Shortly after the passage of the 1938 Act the FDA was moved out of the Department of Agriculture and placed in the Federal Security Agency. This organization later became the Department of Health, Education and Welfare (1953) and then the Department of Health and Human Services (1979). These organizational changes reduced the possibility of regulatory capture by agricultural interests, and placed drug regulation within organizations that were more clearly focused on the health and well-being of citizens.

The next major change in the structure and role of the FDA occurred in 1962, with the Kefauver–Harris amendments to the Act authorizing the existence of the FDA. This amendment was passed in the wake of the thalidomide scandal. Thalidomide was a tranquilizer that was widely used (sold over the counter) in the late 1950s, especially for pregnant women with morning sickness. It became apparent, however, that this drug produced significant birth defects (Botting, 2002). The United States was spared most effects of this disaster because of the work of Dr Frances Kelsey in the FDA, who identified the patterns of birth defects in Europe and prevented approval of the drug.[4]

The Kefauver–Harris amendment established the basics of the regime of drug regulations that exists today. First, there must be proof of efficacy, as well as safety, for a drug to be licensed. That is, the candidate drug must show that it can improve the condition for which it is intended. In addition, the drug must be shown to be safe. Safety is, of course, a relative concept. All drugs will have side-effects, but those side-effects must be sufficiently low that the benefits of the drug outweigh the negative side-effects. Further, those side-effects must be revealed to the patient, and to the physician who prescribes the medication. That disclosure of side-effects was added as one component of a requirement for complete labeling of the drug. Finally, the Act required assessment of over 3,500 drugs that were already on the market, using the same criteria as those applied to new drugs.

After Kefauver–Harris, the powers of the FDA were gradually expanded to cover more areas of healthcare. First came the power to regulate medical devices such as artificial joints and pacemakers. The FDA also gained authority to regulate electromagnetic imaging, for example, X-rays and CAT scans. The regulation of biologics—medications derived from plants or other organisms[5]—was also moved over from Agriculture. Further, the same rules used for drugs came to be applied to the safety of cosmetics. Finally, in 1969, the FDA began surveillance of so-called GRAS (generally recognized as safe) medicines, such as aspirin.

As well as gaining some powers, the FDA has also lost some areas of control over the years. For example, the FDA has lost some of its control over opioids to the Department of Justice, given that these drugs were so readily abused and that legal prescription drugs were being diverted to illegal purposes. The FDA also lost control over pesticides to the Environmental Protection Agency (EPA). While no organization in government likes to lose part of its mandate, these changes have allowed the FDA to focus more clearly on the fundamental mission of regulating pharmaceuticals and food.

The FDA has also gained some regulatory powers, notably over tobacco. The Tobacco Control Act of 2009 gave the agency the ability to control many aspects of the sale of tobacco, although not to ban its sale. As is true for other products regulated by the FDA, tobacco products now had to have complete listings of ingredients. Much of the powers given to the FDA were over the labeling of tobacco products, for example banning terms such as "light" or "mild" that might lead the consumer to believe that some cigarettes were less harmful than others, and banning flavored cigarettes that tended to appeal more to younger people. The same sorts of labeling constraints placed on cigarettes were imposed on smokeless tobacco.

The Act also allowed the FDA to work together with the EPA and the Federal Trade Commission (FTC) to put pressure on the tobacco industry in other ways. The EPA began to take more actions against "secondhand smoke" in the environment, and the FTC looked even harder at tobacco advertising, especially those advertisements that might be especially appealing to young people. The FDA finally banned mentholated cigarettes in 2022, a product that had been especially popular among African-Americans and was thought to contribute to significantly higher rates of smoking in that community than in the rest of the population.

Although it tends to portray itself as an expert, technical organization, the FDA is not immune from political pressures. The political nature of the agency was very clear during the COVID-19 pandemic when it was under pressure to approve vaccines, as well as to approve some less efficacious drugs that were advocated by President Trump and his supporters. In 2022 the FDA came under additional pressure to approve dispensing abortifacients through the mail without a visit to a doctor's office, as a response to the Supreme Court overturning *Roe v Wade* (Belluck, 2021). Also, in 2023 the agency allowed retail pharmacies to dispense the medications, reversing previous requirements for in-person dispensing by physicians (Gonzalez, 2023).

Drug approval process

The process through which new pharmaceuticals are approved for the market is central to understanding how the FDA functions. This process is the means through which a drug company can demonstrate that their product is indeed safe and efficacious. As I will discuss, this process does protect the public, but it is also rather slow, and hence may seem to prevent potentially useful, or even life-saving, drugs from reaching patients as quickly as might be desirable. The vaccines for COVID-19, for example, did not go through the full process before being given an emergency use authorization, after it was clear that there was minimal risk and that the vaccines could prevent infection by the virus. The process for approving a new drug usually goes through the following steps:

(1) The process begins with an investigational new drug (IND) application. After a company has conducted animal testing, or other forms of testing, they can apply for their new drug to be an IND. When the FDA approves the application (based on the evidence from the earlier tests) and it is also approved by the local Institutional Review Body (IRB),[6] it can begin the process of licensing.
(2) Phase 1 Trials. At the first stage a small number (20–80) of human subjects receive the drug. This stage is primarily to evaluate safety, and to identify the most probable side-effects of the drug. These individuals need not suffer from the condition for which the medicine is intended.
(3) Phase 2 Trials. This stage of testing in humans involves much larger numbers of subjects who have the condition for which the drug is being developed.

This stage is typically done as a "double blind" experiment in which neither the patients involved nor the researchers know who has been given the new drug and who is in a control group who are given a placebo. This phase of testing focuses on effectiveness, although it also must be concerned with safety.

(4) Phase 3 Trials. After a meeting between FDA staff and the sponsor of the new drug to plan the trials, Phase 3 trials take place. These may involve thousands of patients, with the trials varying dosages, and administering the drug in combination with other drugs to test for interactions. These tests may also involve different populations (gender, race, age, etc.), although these trials are often criticized for not being sufficiently inclusive.

(5) Review Meeting. After the completion of Phase 3 trials, there is a review meeting between the drug sponsor and the FDA. This meeting involves a discussion of the results of the trials and any issues that may be relevant for further consideration of the drug.

(6) New Drug Application. The drug sponsor then formally asks the FDA to approve the new drug. The application contains all the information from the testing, as well as chemical and pharmaceutical data. These data are reviewed by a team of experts from the FDA, and perhaps also external experts composing an advisory committee for the agency. After the initial application is filed, the FDA has 60 days to decide whether the information is sufficient to proceed with a full review.

(7) Labeling. The FDA reviews the proposed labeling of the new drug, to ensure that the information is complete, and assures that healthcare providers will receive the necessary information if the drug is approved.

(8) Facility Inspection. The FDA inspects the facilities in which the drug will be manufactured.

(9) Approval. If all the steps above meet the standards of safety and efficacy of the new drug, it is approved and can go onto the market.

This is a long process that may take years from the beginning to the end. In some cases, such as the vaccines used in the COVID-19 pandemic, the FDA may issue an "emergency use authorization" to allow drugs to be used when there is no available alternative option and the effects of not making the drugs available are extreme (Krause and Gruber, 2020). During the pandemic, despite the absence of the full authorization of the vaccines, most members of the public were willing to use them, and did so with minimal adverse consequences.

Current challenges in pharmaceutical regulation

Although the basic methodology for reviewing and approving new drugs is in place, there are a number of challenges for the FDA as it attempts to balance pressures coming from the pharmaceutical industry with the demands of the public for safe and effective medications. The danger as seen by the industry is that too strict regulation will kill the goose that has been laying golden eggs for some years, and has made major contributions to improving the health status of Americans. As seen from consumer advocates and some medical practitioners, the danger is that lax regulation will allow dangerous drugs, and some drugs that are unneeded (given the existence of effective, and often lower cost drugs, for the same conditions) into the medical marketplace.

Autonomy

The first and perhaps greatest challenge to the FDA concerns its autonomy from the pharmaceutical industry. A related problem involves the extent to which drug trials are as independent as they should be, or whether they are too heavily influenced by the pharmaceutical industry. This issue arises in part because the pharmaceutical industry is a major lobbyist in Washington, spending more each year for lobbying than almost any other industry. This lobbying is also a major reason that drug prices in the United States continue to be significantly higher than in other countries (even though much of the development of these medicines is done by American firms).

The autonomy of the FDA is threatened by a 1992 Act of Congress that allowed the FDA to collect user fees for the approval process. The Prescription Drug User Fee Act (PDUFA) allows the FDA to collect substantial fees for each new drug that is considered for approval (see Table 6.1). There are also substantially smaller fees when manufacturers of generic drugs want to have their products approved for distribution. The FDA is permitted to use these fees only for supporting the drug approval process, and only so long as it meets certain performance standards, for example the length of time required to review a new drug application. Similar fees are charged for the makers of medical devices.

While these user fees may make good sense as a means of making those who benefit from government services pay for those services (Kitchen et al., 2019), they also run the risk of making the FDA too dependent on "Big Pharma". The pharmaceutical industry depends on the FDA, and could not sell new drugs without going through the approval process, but the FDA may have reasons to approve drugs more readily in order to collect the fees. These close financial connections raise issues of the independence of the agency, and about the safety of the medicines that are approved.

Table 6.1: User fees for drug approval process (in dollars)

	Fiscal Year 2022	Fiscal Year 2021
Requiring Clinical Data	3,117,218	2,875,842
Not Requiring Clinical Data	1,558,609	1,437,981
Program Fee	369,413	336,432
Generic Drug Fee	225,712	196,848

Source: USFDA (2022).

Similar problems of conflicts of interest arise in the advisory committees that are important for the final approval of drugs. Committee members typically are academic physicians and other experts who review the evidence on a candidate drug and advise on its approval. Many of these experts also have connections with the pharmaceutical industry, having performed drug trials for a firm, or perhaps having a financial interest in a firm. There is evidence that these apparent conflicts of interest do indeed influence the voting (Phan-Kanter, 2014). The dilemma is that these are the best people to assess a new drug, given their experience and knowledge of the existing pharmaceuticals for the medical condition in question.

Finally, there are questions concerning the autonomy of actors within clinical trials that are taking place in medical schools or hospitals. First, to what extent do the medical professionals who lead the drug trials have real autonomy? Performing these trials through grants, whether from the drug companies themselves or government sources, is important to their standing in the profession, and perhaps also to their income. They therefore do not want to offend the pharmaceutical companies with too many negative findings (Allman, 2003). In addition, there are populations of individuals who are always ready to consent to take part in trials, perhaps because of their need for an income. This raises questions about the meaning of informed consent (Fisher, 2007), as well as about the validity of findings on individuals who have participated in multiple trials.

There are several policy options for addressing these questions of autonomy of drug trials. The most obvious is to have the trials funded and managed by the FDA, rather than through the drug companies themselves. Assuming this responsibility would add millions to the annual budget of the FDA, and would therefore require larger user fees, or higher appropriations from Congress. Another alternative to direct funding by the firms would be for the pharmaceutical manufacturers to create a foundation or other non-profit organization that would fund and manage the trials. Either of these options would still require cooperation from hospitals and medical schools, so may not be a fool-proof alternative.

Post-approval controls

The major emphasis of reviewing new pharmaceuticals within the FDA is during the pre-approval stage. The clinical trials and the other components of the review process are designed to ensure that drugs that reach the public are safe and efficacious. Despite all the research and analysis that goes into the approval process, some medicines that are not safe do reach the marketplace, and do cause harm to patients. The most commonly cited example of this negative outcome was Vioxx, a drug approved in 1999 for chronic pain associated with arthritis. After approval, it became clear that the drug significantly increased the probability of heart attacks and strokes, and the drug was voluntarily removed from the market in 2004 (Nesi, 2008).[7]

The Vioxx experience demonstrated the need for more continuous monitoring of drugs after approval. The major instrument utilized by the FDA for these purposes is the FDA Adverse Events Reporting System (FAERS). This system is particularly designed to collect evidence of "serious adverse events", such as death or injuries that would cause disability. In addition, there are some post-marketing studies done through a system called REMS (Risk Evaluation and Mitigation Strategy) initiated in 2007 by the FDA amendments passed that year. As the name implies, this system focuses on the risks of adverse reactions and the means of reducing the impact of those reactions.

Despite the various detection and remediation systems that are now in place, there are still numerous complaints about the side-effects of many drugs on the market. For example, the antibiotic ciprofloxacin has been cited a number of times as having serious side-effects, especially for older patients. Despite the complaints, the FDA has allowed the drug to remain on the market (Khazan, 2021). The severe reactions have occurred in a relatively small number of cases, and the drug does work for many infections, so the decision has been to let it continue to be sold.

Advertising

Pharmaceutical companies spend a vast amount of money on advertising. They have been advertising to physicians for some years, but the FDA first allowed drug companies to advertise directly to the public in 1997. Since that time spending has grown significantly, and in 2020 it is estimated that "Big Pharma" spent over $6.5 billion on advertising to the general public (Statista, 2022), mostly for ads on television but also in magazines (especially those directed to senior citizens). This spending was up from $3.9 billion in 2012.

Several issues arise from this high level of advertising drugs to patients. The first is simply that this amount of money is being added to the costs of pharmaceuticals, so the medicines that patients need will be more expensive. Indeed, one study found that many of the major drug manufacturers were spending more on advertising than they were on research and development (AHIP, 2021).[8] Whenever their profit levels are questioned by Congress or the public, the drug companies always justify them by spending on research and development, but advertising is also adding to the prices paid by consumers, and by health insurers.

The second issue that arises from the high levels of advertising by drug firms is that it creates demand for certain drugs, and places pressures on doctors to prescribe them. A patient may see an advertisement for a new drug that is alleged to produce wonderful results for the condition from which the patient suffers. The patient then asks their doctor for the advertised treatment, and may be unhappy if the doctor refuses. That refusal may be because of the potential dangers of the drug, the fact that its performance is no better than an older, less-expensive drug, or perhaps other reasons. Whatever the reason the physician is placed in an awkward situation, especially when there is increased emphasis on measuring patient satisfaction (see Chapter 9).

From some available evidence doctors are not as quick as the pharmaceutical manufacturers might like to respond to requests from patients for drugs they have

Table 6.2: Doctors' responses to requests for medications seen in advertisements (answers from patients)

Recommended Lifestyle or Behavioral Changes	15%
Recommended a Different Prescription Drug	14%
Recommended the Requested Drug	12%
Recommended an Over-the-Counter Drug	11%
Other, No Response	48%

Source: Kaiser Family Foundation, *Health Tracking Poll*, October 14–20, 2015.

seen advertised on television. In one study by the Kaiser Family Foundation (see Table 6.2) it was found that only about one doctor in nine was responsive to the requests of patients for a drug they had seen advertised. A larger number of the patients reported that doctors offered other treatments, including lifestyle changes, rather than opting for a new medication.

As important as drug advertising to the public is as a regulatory issue, advertising to doctors may be even more important. It is, in the end, doctors that have the authority to write prescriptions. Further, patients may be even more likely to follow the advice of their physician on drugs than they would to accept the pitches made to them in advertisements (Frosch et al., 2010). If a pharmaceutical company can convince physicians that their new drug is superior to those already on the market, they are more likely to be successful in selling that drug than they could be by emphasizing advertisements to the general public.

Drug companies have been involved with advertising to physicians for decades, but the issues about the possible undue influence of that advertising have become more publicized over the past decade. Calling some of the attempts of drug companies to influence doctors "advertising" is to be excessively generous. In addition to information about new drugs, doctors may receive dinners, vacations and a plethora of other benefits (Table 6.3) from the pharmaceutical companies. Discussions of the influence of these contacts between physicians and drug companies has been the source of a new round of "muckraking" about the drug industry (Angell, 2009; Goldacre, 2014).

In fairness, it is not only the advertising by the pharmaceutical companies that is causing problems with the use and abuse of prescription medicines. The internet has become a major source of information and disinformation about medications, comparable perhaps to the situation existing prior to the licensing of drugs. This problem became very evident during the COVID-19 pandemic when a number of medications, most notably a veterinary medicine used for parasites in horses, were touted as cures for the virus. For some reason, many individuals appeared more willing to accept uncorroborated information from the internet than they were the advice of medical professionals.

While the above case of drug use and abuse is particularly egregious, there have been a number of instances in which the "off-label" use of drugs has been

Table 6.3: Frequency of physician–drug company interactions (percentage of respondents)

Receive Gifts	83
Receive Drug Samples	78
Reimbursements	35
Payments for Consulting	18
Speaker's Fees	16
Payments for Serving on Advisory Board	9
Payments for Enrolling Patients in Clinical Trials	3
Any of the Above Relationships	94

Source: Campbell (2007).

promoted, some producing substantial harm to the users. Although drugs are licensed for a particular use, off-label use is not strictly illegal, and in some cases may be efficacious for the patient and supported by medical practitioners. The need is to find a policy solution that can balance needs for safety and efficacy of medications with the opportunities for innovation (Stafford, 2012). For example, the FDA could require post-marketing information from doctors about off-label use of drugs, or create data resources for reporting on uses and problems with this practice, a practice that could be facilitated by greater use of electronic health records.

Orphan drugs

The discussion concerning the process for evaluating drugs by the FDA assumes that drug companies are anxious to get the medication into the market. That is usually a good assumption, but in some cases it is not true. It has been difficult to get drug companies interested in developing medications for illnesses that affect a relatively small number of people. These drugs will take as long to develop as do other drugs, but can be expected to yield very little revenue. The only way these drugs could be profitable would be if their costs to the patient were extremely high, and then many insurance companies would not be willing to pay for them.

The 1983 Orphan Drug Act allowed the FDA to assist in the development and use of these so-called "orphan drugs". If the FDA recognizes that the drug is indeed directed at a rare condition, and some drug company is willing to function as a sponsor (Davies et al., 2017), the company involved is eligible for benefits such as tax credits for the clinical trials, exemption from user fees and a potential several years of market exclusivity once the drug is approved. Further, once the review process is initiated, it is much simpler than that required for most drugs, in part because the possibilities of random trials are limited because of the small population of patients (see Box 6.1). Given the economic issues involved with those drugs with a limited market, in extreme cases the FDA has the capacity to create a "state-owned enterprise" to manufacture the drug. These benefits are substantial, but may still be insufficient to get a drug company to make the investments required.

Box 6.1: Fast-tracking drugs

What is fast tracking?

A more frequent and open communication between the developers and the FDA, which accelerates the approval process and provides closer attention. Drug companies can request fast-track designation, and the request can occur at any time during the drug development process. Upon receipt, the FDA will review the fast-track designation request and make a decision within 60 days.

Method/how

Fast-track is a process designed to facilitate and advance the review of drugs that treat serious conditions and fill unmet medical needs, based on promising animal or human data. Fast-tracking can get important new drugs to the patient earlier.

How to qualify for fast-tracking

Any drug being developed to treat or prevent a condition with no current therapy obviously is directed at an unmet need. If there are available therapies, a fast-track drug must show some advantage over available therapy, such as:

(1) Superior effectiveness
(2) Avoiding serious side-effects of an available therapy
(3) Improving the diagnosis of a serious condition where early diagnosis results in an improved outcome
(4) Decreasing clinically significant toxicity of an available therapy
(5) Ability to address emerging or anticipated public health needs.

After the drug is approved

The drug is now eligible for more frequent meetings with FDA officials to discuss the drug's development; more frequent written communication with the FDA; accelerated approval and priority review; rolling review.

The "orphan drug" issue is in at least one way now becoming more common in American healthcare. As physicians become capable of developing treatments tailored to the specific genetic makeup of individuals and the specific nature of their disease (usually cancer) drugs may have a market of only one person. These developments may pose more problems for the insurance companies than they do for the FDA, but for the FDA there is a question of whether each individual's drug needs to be licensed, or only the class of drugs.

Antibiotics

Although antibiotics are one of the most commonly used class of drugs, there are significant problems with the available drugs on the market. Many of these drugs have been used for a number of years and microbes have become resistant to them. There are some microbes now that are resistant to all known antibiotics,[9] and that problem is likely to get worse given the widespread use, and abuse, of antibiotics (see Pierre and Carelli, 2022). Given that many individuals do not take the full course of antibiotics when prescribed, the microbes that survive develop a resistance to the antibiotics.

Why, when so many people require antibiotics (approximately 250 million prescriptions are written for antibiotics in the United States each year), are drug companies reluctant to engage in research for new antibiotics? As is true for most things in the pharmaceutical industry, the answer is money (see Shlaes and Bradford, 2018). Drugs for diseases such as diabetes, arthritis and other chronic diseases have to be bought year after year as long as the patient lives. Antibiotics generally are taken for a week or two, the infection is overcome, and there is no more need for the antibiotics to be bought until there is another infection. In short, the big money in pharmaceuticals is in chronic diseases. This is especially true as the American population ages and suffers from more chronic conditions.

The FDA has not been passive when considering the absence of new antibiotics coming onto the market. The agency began around the beginning of the twenty-first century to consider the problem of antimicrobial resistance (Rodriguez-Rojas et al., 2013) and to develop strategies for coping with this problem. It has also sponsored programs directed at finding new antibiotics in soils and plants. But even with those efforts there are an increasing number of cases of patients dying because a bacterial infection cannot be treated. The pharmaceutical companies still have less incentive to develop new antibiotics than they do to develop treatments for arthritis or heart disease that a patient may take for many years.

Dietary supplements

Food supplements, or dietary supplements, are a major business in the United States,[10] and they are often marketed as a "natural" alternative to the drugs that are regulated by the FDA. The manufacturers and their supporters often make extravagant claims about the capacity of these supplements to reduce symptoms of medical problems (although rarely are claims made about curing the problems). Although these supplements are treated like medicines in many ways, and are regularly sold in drug stores along with regulated drugs, the FDA has little control over them (Starr, 2015). There are controls over the adulteration of the supplements and the cleanliness of the production facilities, but little else.

The food supplement industry has faced other forms of regulation, especially over claims that may be made about their effectiveness. The FTC (generally responsible for false advertising) has engaged in some regulatory actions over advertising, but the advertising is often sufficiently vague that it is difficult to prove outright deception. State governments, usually through their attorneys general, have also been active in regulating this industry and attempting to rein in any excessive claims that may discourage patients from getting more effective treatments.

Tobacco

The FDA has been empowered to regulate tobacco products, but has done so rather slowly and seemingly ineffectively. For example, it took several years for the agency to issue final rules regulating flavored cigarettes, which were known to be how many teenagers became addicted to tobacco. More recently, its regulation of the e-cigarette and vaping industries has been weak (Florko and Welle, 2022). The agency's primary mission has been the regulation of the pharmaceutical industry, and regulating tobacco seems to require rather different procedures, for example there is no need for clinical trials, and it falls outside the expertise of many of the members of the organization.

More inclusive testing

Not all medications will be effective for all people, and it is important to gain as much of that information as possible from the testing that is done before the approval of drugs. One of the potentially important omissions in drug trials is children, and much of the advertising for drugs that appears on television and elsewhere points out that the medication is not in fact approved for children. While some might be inappropriate for children in any case, some are potentially useful, and more inclusive testing might make it possible to prescribe those drugs.

As well as having very few trials of new medicines done on children, women also tend to make up a relatively small proportion of test subjects. For both children and women, part of the reluctance to include more in the samples is some fear of adverse effects, and potential suits. Women involved in a drug trial may be pregnant or become pregnant during the trial, with possible harm to the fetus. Likewise, few researchers would want to risk harm to children, even though the medication may be potentially beneficial to young people. Finally, there is often a racial imbalance in testing and, although some medical specialties are eliminating any mention of race in treatment protocols, there are still questions about inclusion in testing (National Academies of Sciences, Engineering, and Medicine, 2022).

Public confidence

A final problem for the FDA is some decline in public confidence in their capacity to ensure a flow of safe and effective medications for patients. There has been a general decline in public confidence in the public sector in the United States, but the decline in confidence in the FDA has been particularly steep. This organization had gained substantial power by demonstrating its expertise and developing a reputation as being competent (Carpenter, 2010). In the 1970s almost three-quarters of the American population had confidence in the FDA, but by 2021 this had shrunk to 37 percent (Robert Wood Johnson Foundation and Chan School of Public Health, 2021). This slip in confidence mirrored a general decline in public health institutions during the pandemic.

The decline in confidence in the FDA had, however, begun before the pandemic. Problems with drugs such as Vioxx that had been approved by the agency were part of the problem, along with the beginning of the anti-vaccination movement against vaccinations such as measles and mumps. Also, the agency was often perceived to be too slow in responding to the needs of the public for new drugs. These possibly contradictory assessments of the FDA had produced sagging confidence before the anti-science and anti-vax elements of the populist movement further undermined its work.

Other dimensions of regulation

While the regulation of pharmaceuticals is the major regulatory aspect of health policy in the United States, there are other dimensions that are significant as well. To some extent regulatory programs are also discussed when discussing broader issues such as cost control and quality, and I will attempt to avoid repetition. That said, however, there will inevitably be some overlap as I focus on regulatory policies, given that the intentions of the regulations are often to reduce cost or increase access.

Certificate of need

Healthcare facilities are very expensive to open and maintain and, as part of the attempt to reduce costs and improve quality, the state of New York initiated a program called "certificate of need", requiring approval of the state government before new facilities could be built. In 1974 the National Health Planning and Resource Development Act made this program national, under the direction of the Department of Housing and Urban Development,[11] although it was to be administered by the states. The Act was repealed in 1986, but many states continued to enforce certificate of need programs. As of 2022, 35 states have functioning certificate of need programs.

Those 35 states use different criteria for need, and also require certification of need for different types of activities. Some may require a certificate for any capital expansion, while others may focus more closely on building new hospitals (especially in areas that are already well-served with hospital beds). For-profit hospitals may not be covered in some states. Even with these variations, the program has had some beneficial effects in reducing excess capacity.[12] That said, however, these programs may produce some negative consequences, especially when there are population shifts and construction of medical facilities does not keep pace with the changing needs of the population.

Regulating facilities

In addition to regulations about the construction of healthcare facilities, there are regulations about their management and the services they deliver. These regulations are becoming more important because of changes in the population, and changes in the manner in which health services are delivered. First, as the population continues to age, the need for long-term care facilities continues to increase. These facilities require substantial regulation to ensure patient safety and the quality of care, especially given the vulnerability of many of the patients. There are also a set of rights for patients in these facilities that help to regulate the behaviors of management and staff.

The other facilities that require a closer look from a regulatory perspective are the increasing number of "urgicare" and ambulatory surgery centers (ASCs). These facilities operate outside of hospitals, and provide some basic medical services in the case of the urgicare centers, and elective surgery in the case of the ASCs. At present, the principal means of regulation of these facilities is through Medicare certification, as well as some state regulations (McGuire, 2013). The problem is perhaps most acute for the ASCs because, although most of the surgeries performed in these centers are considered routine, there is still the problem of complications that the centers do not have the staff or equipment to handle.

Regulating health insurance

Private health insurance is the dominant means through which Americans receive coverage for healthcare. This insurance is regulated by the states in a number of ways, including the premiums that can be charged, and the manner in which benefits are determined, and the relationships with providers. Almost all private health insurance is organized on a state-by-state basis, in part because of the differences in regulations in the 50 states.[13]

The federal government has also become involved in regulating health insurance. The Health Insurance Portability and Accountability Act of 1996 (HIPAA) provides some national regulations on health insurance, as well as limits on the dissemination of patient information by health providers. One problem with group health insurance provided by employers has been that if the individual moved from one job to another they might lose health coverage, especially for pre-existing conditions. This problem within the market locked many workers—especially those with conditions such as diabetes or cancer—into jobs when they might have been able to get better jobs but would not be covered against major illnesses.

HIPAA essentially guaranteed any new employees coverage under an employer's health plan after 18 months, and reduced the time without coverage by the time they had had "credible coverage" under another plan before they made the move to the new job. Credible coverage has been deemed to mean coverage under another employer's plan, or Medicaid or Medicare, or an individual plan covering the pre-existing condition. This eligibility for coverage is valid for general health insurance, but coverage for specialized treatments such as vision or dental can be more restrictive.

While HIPAA is important for protecting individual privacy and the confidentiality of medical records, it can also pose some problems within the medical care system. Some privacy advocates have been concerned that the movement to electronic health records, which can save money and improve the quality of care, will also lead to greater ease in disseminating information about patients. In addition, the restrictions in HIPAA have made some aspects of medical research more difficult (Gostin and Nass, 2009).

The federal government also regulates access to health insurance through the Comprehensive Budget Reconciliation Act (COBRA), which was passed during the Reagan administration. In addition to the capacity to move between employers and retain coverage, COBRA allows individuals who lose coverage after leaving a job to retain coverage in the group for at least some limited (and variable) time period. This opportunity also applies to families when the covered employee passes away, and to some other "events". When the right to continue coverage in a group plan is invoked, the individual will be responsible for paying the full cost of the program, so that after the passage of the Affordable Care Act there may be more affordable options available.

Regulating the health professions

Finally, there are some regulations used to attempt to control the medical professions. Most of the controls on doctors and nurses, however, are in the form of incentives rather than regulations—for example, bonuses from Medicaid and Medicare for doctors working in poorer communities. Although it is hoped that financial incentives will help to do things such as move more doctors into general practice, or get more practitioners working in underserved areas, these have not been nearly as effective as the incentives operating in the market that tell doctors to become surgeons, and to locate in urban areas.

Licensing, including the capacity to revoke licenses, is the primary means of regulating the health professions (see Chapter 9). This licensure is conducted primarily at the state level, and includes not only doctors and nurses but also, depending upon the state, a number of other health professionals. In addition, medical laboratories and testing facilities are licensed or accredited. While this level of control appears impressive, it is important to remember that a good deal of this activity is self-regulation by the professions. Medical associations are given the right to license and to sanction medical care providers in the name of the government, and governments tend to rely heavily on the expertise of the associations. While this makes sense in terms of not developing a large expert staff to oversee licensing, it does provide the medical professions a great deal of autonomy when dealing with their patients.

Conclusion

There is a significant regulatory dimension to health policy in the United States, much of it oriented toward the safety and efficacy of medicine. The centrality of pharmaceutical regulation is in part a function of the importance of drugs in contemporary healthcare—the average American over age 70, for example, takes four medicines each day, and one-third take five or more per day. The centrality of drug regulation is also in part a function of the size and importance of "Big Pharma" as an industry, and as a lobbyist in Washington and in state capitols. Although the FDA has been a well-respected organization for most of its existence, recent events (including the COVID-19 pandemic) have undermined public confidence to some extent, and it is important that the agency rebuild that trust.

Pharmaceuticals are not the only targets for regulatory activity, and some of these additional regulatory policies, for example those directed at health insurance and the medical professions, have been discussed in this chapter. Other aspects of regulation are, however, also discussed in the chapters on cost and quality. This division of the discussion of regulation was made in order to better explain those very basic aspects of health policy. Regulation as a policy instrument is important, but more important are the effects of regulation on improving quality and lowering costs.

7

Access to healthcare

For Americans confronting their healthcare system the most pressing single issue is access. If people cannot visit doctors, go to hospitals, get their prescriptions filled or get any other needed health services, then all the high-tech medical facilities that exist in the United States are of little use to them. The sad news is that for many Americans access is very limited, even after the passage of the Affordable Care Act (ACA) and other reforms of the health system. Each year millions of Americans do not receive adequate treatment for health conditions, and are concerned about their capacity to pay for such medical care as they are able to obtain.

As should be obvious by this point in the book, the major impediment to access for Americans is money. Programs such as Medicaid, Medicare, the Children's Health Insurance Program (CHIP) and the ACA all attempt to provide healthcare to citizens at no cost, or at lower costs than they might otherwise confront in the marketplace. However, even with these programs, there are economic barriers for many Americans seeking medical care. For example, the co-pays and deductibles in Medicare are not inconsequential amounts of money for retirees on fixed income, or for someone in a low wage job. And the insurance offered under the ACA requires the insured person to pay premiums, even if they are subsidized, and also has deductibles and co-pays. In addition, for individuals who receive health insurance through their employer, the costs of premiums and co-pays has been increasing (see Table 7.1 and Chapter 8). Even if insured, individuals have to make economic choices about healthcare that can reduce their effective access to services.

But not all the barriers to healthcare are economic. There are a number of geographical, social and cultural barriers, all of which can reduce the ability of citizens, even those with insurance and without economic problems, from receiving the type of care they need. Further, these non-economic barriers may be even more difficult to confront effectively than are the economic ones. Any government willing to spend the money can eliminate economic barriers to accessing care, but many of the other sources of poor access will remain, and will continue to produce inequalities in the ways in which people consume healthcare in the United States.

The structure of the healthcare system in the United States itself—the jungle nature of the system—also tends to constrain access to healthcare. To get access the patient must know how to deal with the insurance companies, the doctors, the hospitals and all the other providers. For routine care, for example visiting a primary care physician (PCP), this may not be too confusing. However, to cope with more serious and extended care dealing with the rules of these various actors—perhaps especially the insurance companies—can take hours of time and a great deal of energy. These problems have become even greater as medical providers contract out services in order to save cost. Even public sector providers

Table 7.1: Decline of individuals receiving insurance through employers (in percentage)

1988	2000	2005	2010	2015	2018	2020
67.3	66.1	62.5	56.3	57.5	58.3	49.4

Source: Kaiser Family Foundation, *Employer Health Benefits Survey*, various years.

such as Medicaid may now use several layers of contractors to reduce their costs, while at the same time causing major difficulties for the insured (Wolfson, 2021).

Economic barriers

Even with a significant public sector presence in health policy there are major economic barriers to access to medical care. Most importantly, there are still a significant number of people in the country who do not have medical insurance. Before the beginning of the COVID-19 pandemic in 2020 approximately 10 percent of the population did not have health insurance. That number increased significantly during the pandemic as thousands of people who lost their jobs lost their employer-provided health insurance. For example, the Commonwealth Fund estimates that as many as 14.6 million workers and their families may have lost employee-sponsored insurance during the pandemic (Fronstin and Woodbury, 2020).[1]

Over time those individuals and families who lost insurance could become eligible for Medicaid, but for some months they were without insurance. Even after the worst of the pandemic appears to have passed, the number of insured persons has not increased as much as might have been expected. Fewer employers who are not required to by the ACA are now offering insurance, and the number of people in stable, full-time jobs has not returned to pre-pandemic levels. Although the pandemic may have made the need for health insurance even more clear to most people, their economic circumstances may make buying the insurance difficult.

The extent to which Americans are uninsured is affected by a number of factors. Income is perhaps the most obvious. As might be expected, the most affluent segments of the population (see Table 7.2) are the most likely to be covered, with very few people having incomes over 400 percent of the poverty level ($104,800) not being covered by insurance, with some of the small number without insurance being self-insured. Despite the existence of Medicaid and CHIP, those below the federal poverty level have the lowest levels of coverage. A good deal of this low rate of insurance is because of the absence of stable addresses, or the capacity to fill out the forms required.

However, many people between the federal poverty level and 200 percent of that amount—the "working poor"—also have low levels of insurance.[2] This group may earn too much to be eligible for Medicaid, is not covered by employer-provided insurance, but may not earn enough to purchase private insurance (even when subsidized through the ACA). The "working poor" are,

Table 7.2: Uninsured by income, age and race (2020)

	Percentage Uninsured
Total Population	8.6
Income	
Below Poverty Level	17.2
0–100 Percent of Poverty	15.0
200–299 Percent of Poverty	11.9
300–399 Percent of Poverty	8.9
400+ Percent of Poverty	3.4
Age	
Under 19	5.6
19–34	14.3
35–44	12.4
45–64	9.6
65+	1.0
Race and Ethnicity	
White, Non-Hispanic	5.4
Asian	5.8
Black	10.4
Hispanic	18.3
Residence	
Medicaid Expansion State	6.4
Non-Expansion State	12.6

Source: US Bureau of the Census, *Health Insurance Coverage in the United States, 2020*, https://www.census.gov/library/publications/2023/demo/p60-281.html.

to a great extent, the component of the population that has the most persistent barriers to gaining access to healthcare. The expansion of Medicaid as a part of the ACA was meant to deal with that problem, but the lack of action by some states and the continuing increases in insurance prices have made solving the problem more difficult.

Absolute levels of income are important for explaining who has health insurance and who does not, but the nature of the employment also matters. If an individual works for government, or for a larger employer in the private sector, the probabilities are good that they will have health insurance as a benefit of employment. Individuals working for small businesses, or who work in the "gig economy", are less likely to have insurance unless they pay for it entirely themselves. Younger workers who move from job to job for short periods are especially unlikely to have health insurance (Tran and Sokas, 2017).

Although working for a large employer may enhance one's chances of having health insurance, those employers are reducing their commitments to providing insurance. As shown in Table 7.1 the proportion of individuals in the United States who have health insurance from their employers has declined from over two-thirds of the population to less than one-half. This reflects, among other things, the declining workforces of traditional large employers—especially manufacturing—as a proportion of all employment, the decline of unionization, increased unemployment during the pandemic and cost reductions by employers. Some of that loss of insurance from employers has been taken up by insurance through the ACA, but the insured are now paying all the bill (after any subsidies from government), rather than having the employer pay most of the bill as in the past.

Further, employers have been shifting more of the costs of health insurance programs they provide to the employees (see Table 7.3). The employees' share of health insurance premiums has been increasing, as have co-pays and deductibles. Therefore, even if an individual does have health insurance, the amount they have to pay out of pocket has continued to increase, and this may deter them from getting all the medical care they need. The increases in payments by the insured have been especially high for family plans.

Age is a second important factor in defining levels of coverage of health insurance. Medicare provides coverage for almost all the population aged 65 and over (Table 7.2). But, even then, some economic factors may intervene to limit coverage. As already noted, Medicare is not inexpensive, and the premiums, co-payments and deductibles can amount to a significant portion of the income of an individual on a fixed income (see Chapter 3). At the other end of the age spectrum, children 19 and under tend to be better insured than does the working age group. Again, public insurance—CHIP—is the principal reason that children who might not otherwise be covered are insured.

Race and ethnicity play a role in the level of insurance coverage in the United States. As might be expected (see Table 7.2) non-Hispanic whites have the highest level of health insurance coverage, followed closely by Asian Americans. Hispanic Americans, on the other hand, had the lowest level of insurance, following

Table 7.3: Cost-shifting to employees by employers (in percentage)

	Employer Subsidy	Employee Contribution	Out of Pocket
2020	7.7	7.4	8.6
2017	4.8	8.0	8.0
2014	5.0	8.5	7.3
2010	5.4	14.7	5.4
2005	11.3	5.6	6.0

Source: Kaiser Family Foundation, annual *Employer Health Benefit Survey*, https://www.census.gov/library/publications/2023/demo/p60-281.html.

African-Americans. The lower levels of coverage for Hispanics may be a function of immigration status and the inability to get coverage from public programs. These differences could be anticipated, given the generally lower access of Black people and other minorities to healthcare, but these differences appear little changed after the implementation of the ACA and other public programs.

Finally, there were marked differences in health insurance coverage between states that had expanded Medicaid under the ACA and those that had not. Almost half as many people lacked coverage in expansion states than in the non-expansion states. The failure to accept the incentives offered by the ACA for expanding Medicaid was clearly a political and ideological decision by state governments, mostly in the South and Midwest, but referendums in a number of these states are forcing governments to accept the expansion, and levels of insurance should increase (see Chapter 4).

Although insurance coverage is important, it does not guarantee that the economic barriers to access will be removed entirely for the individual and their family. Not all insurance plans provided to individuals, even through employers or through approved ACA plans, remove economic barriers to access. There are very few "first dollar" coverage programs available in the private marketplace, meaning that individuals have to pay co-pays and deductibles to use their insurance, and the premiums for those policies are very high. Therefore, the insured individual is confronted with a decision of whether they really need to visit the doctor or whether it is better to hold on to their cash.

Not all health insurance is the same, and many people who are now insured have inadequate insurance, or policies that have extremely high deductibles and co-payments. The Trump administration issued regulations that made policies with very high deductibles, and that covered relatively few aspects of medical care, available under the ACA. These policies would meet the requirements for declaring a person to be insured under the ACA, but they mean that the individuals "covered" under these policies face extremely large economic barriers when seeking medical care (Rabin et al., 2020). The health insurance market has long offered catastrophic policies that tended to be bought by relatively young people who wanted some protection in case of accidents or severe illnesses, but these have become a larger segment of the insurance market.

Leaving aside the effects of the Trump administration on insurance coverage through the ACA, a significant percentage of Americans are underinsured, even if they have health insurance (Box 7.1). One estimate is that over 12 percent of the population has insurance that has high deductibles, inadequate coverage or both (Collins et al., 2020). Other estimates are that 43 percent of the population is underinsured (Commonwealth Fund, 2022b). Individuals may purchase policies that provide limited benefits—usually only for catastrophic illness or injury—for much less than the cost of comprehensive coverage. For many young people who think that the probabilities of their falling ill is low, and who have limited income, these minimal coverage plans appear to make a good deal of sense.

Box 7.1: What is underinsurance?

A person is underinsured if:

(1) Out-of-pocket costs for healthcare over the prior 12 months, excluding premiums, are 10 percent or more of household income; or

(2) Out-of-pocket costs for healthcare over the prior 12 months, excluding premiums, are 5 percent or more of household income if income is under 200 percent of the federal poverty line; or

(3) Deductibles for health insurance are over 5 percent of household income.

Source: Collins et al. (2017).

The minimalist policies may appear to make sense, until the poorly insured person falls ill, and must pay a significant amount of money out of pocket, perhaps enough to bankrupt them (Woolhandler and Himmelstein, 2013). And to some extent the effects of underinsurance on access are identical to those of no insurance. An individual who is facing high deductibles and co-payments is not as likely to seek medical care as someone who has insurance with more modest out-of-pocket costs. The reluctance to get medical care is likely to be especially true for screening and preventative care, which in turn may lead to higher costs (for the individual and for society as a whole) in the long run.

During the COVID-19 pandemic, and then probably beyond, another economic barrier to access has become important. A good deal of healthcare, especially visits with PCPs, has been delivered through "telemedicine" over the internet. If, however, one does not have good access to the internet then the choice became whether to take risks and see a physician in person, or not get any care at all. The success of this form of health delivery during the pandemic crisis means that the future of healthcare may also depend on reliable access to telecommunications (Sieck et al., 2021).

Finally, the nature of work itself, as well as the level of income earned, may constitute another economic barrier to access to healthcare. For someone in a white-collar occupation, there is generally little problem taking a few hours off to go to an appointment with a physician. If, however, the individual is in a blue-collar job, paid by the hour, that may not be so easy, and may result in losing some hours of pay. Some PCPs have office hours outside normal working hours, but most specialists do not, so the patient must take time off from work to make the visit to the provider. Further, for people (usually women) who are primary caregivers for children, or elderly family members, or both, getting time away to tend to their own medical issues may be extremely difficult.

In summary, the United States spends a huge amount of money on medical care, but money is still a barrier to access for many citizens. Indeed, it remains the most significant barrier to access for many people. Even for individuals insured by the insurance programs offered by government there are economic barriers. These are perhaps especially high in Medicare for retirees living on fixed incomes. The improvements in economic access provided through the ACA have made an impact, but many Americans still do without healthcare, or face debt or bankruptcy when they do have to consume medical services.

Race

Access to medical care in the United States is also very much affected by race. To some extent the race dimension of exclusion from access overlaps with the economic one, given that average per capita income of African-Americans is 61 percent of that of white Americans, and income for Hispanics averages 74 percent (US Bureau of the Census, 2022).[3] But the racial disparities cannot be explained entirely by economics, and factors associated directly with race have an independent impact on disparities in insurance coverage as well as use of, and outcomes of, medical services.

African-Americans are significantly less covered by health insurance than are whites and Asian-Americans. Even after the expansion of Medicaid in many states, and the availability of relatively lower cost insurance through the ACA, African-Americans are less insured, even when levels of income are taken into account. Some of this difference may reflect the structure of employment, with African-Americans less likely to work for employers who provide benefits like health insurance. And it may also reflect lower levels of information about health insurance options in poor and minority communities (Lillie-Blanton and Hoffman, 2005), especially after the adoption of the ACA.

Americans of Hispanic origin tend to have even lower levels of coverage by health insurance than do African-Americans. They face many of the same economic and information barriers as do African-Americans, but may have two additional barriers. One is that a number of Hispanic residents are in the United States without documents, and therefore are not eligible for public programs such as Medicaid or the ACA. A few cities, for example Los Angeles, do provide free medical care to undocumented residents, but the majority are excluded. Although they would be provided services, undocumented residents tend to use emergency rooms less than do other residents because of fear of being found out and deported (Wallace, 2012).

In addition to the difficulties in access experienced by minority group members, the telecommunications issues already mentioned may further complicate their capacity to cope with the healthcare system. Individuals who have less access to telecommunications, either because of cost, no available services, or lack of knowledge do not have the capacity to get health information and advice online. While in some instances this may protect them from misinformation, for example from the anti-vaxxers, it also denies people of potentially useful information.

Although there are important barriers to access to medical care facing minority groups in the contemporary healthcare system, there are also longer-term forces that diminish the use of healthcare. For African-Americans, the history of neglect and abuse by the healthcare system produces distrust in the present day. The most famous example of the abuses was the Tuskegee syphilis experiment (Reverby, 2000; Corbie-Smith, 1999), but there have been other abuses that have tended to drive people toward self-care, or toward using advice and support from their community. This pattern has been evident recently in the large number of African-Americans who have been reluctant to be vaccinated against COVID-19, although there are also some more specific concerns about the vaccine (Gamble, 2021).[4]

The evidence is rather clear that members of minority groups in the United States (with perhaps the exception of Asian-Americans) do not have as good access to medical care, or as good outcomes from the healthcare system, as do white Americans. Some of the barriers encountered are economic, but others have to do with implicit and explicit biases within the system. Although there have been continuing attempts to address these biases in the delivery system, the evidence is largely that there has been relatively little change (Dovido et al., 2016). The racial disparities in outcomes and in satisfaction with the system persist.

Gender

Gender also poses access problems for healthcare. Some of these problems are related directly to how the healthcare system treats women, but others are a function of economic and social factors that indirectly affect access. To deal with those indirect, largely economic, influences first, one of the major factors is that women tend to be in more low-paying positions in the economy than are men, and therefore often do not have employer-provided insurance. The "glitch" in ACA insurance (see Chapter 5) also means that families are not as likely to be covered as the employee, and this design problem in the program can affect women not working outside the home.

There are also a number of factors at work within the healthcare system itself. Studies have found that, regardless of income, education or race, women tend not to receive as much attention within the system as do men (Cameron et al., 2010). Also, there are declining numbers of doctors specializing in obstetrics and gynecology, in part because of the threats of malpractice suits and the high premiums for malpractice (Hollowell, 2023). Also, the standard assumptions about how some diseases, notably heart disease, present are based on male patients and therefore women may be misdiagnosed and not receive adequate care (Stefanick, 2017). This list could be extended, but the fundamental point is that the healthcare system in the United States does not provide equal access for women.

Geography

It matters for access to healthcare not only how much money you earn, your race and your education, but also where you live. In the United States there

Table 7.4: Distribution of physicians by state (2020, active physicians per 100,000 population)

	High		Low
District of Columbia	871.0	Idaho	196.1
Massachusetts	466.0	Mississippi	196.6
Maryland	393.5	Oklahoma	209.6
New York	389.4	Wyoming	211.7
Vermont	386.2	Arkansas	215.4

Source: American Medical Colleges, *Physician Workforce Data Report*, 2022.

are marked differences in access to medical facilities and practitioners based on the state in which a person lives, whether they live in an urban or rural area, or what neighborhood in a city they live in. These are not minor differences and, if anything, the differences are increasing. Access to healthcare, especially in rural areas, has been declining for some years, and appears likely to continue to decline without significant intervention by government.

We can begin to examine these differences by looking at the availability of physicians across the 50 states and the District of Columbia (Table 7.4). The District is the best served area in the country, followed by states such as Massachusetts, Maryland and Vermont. Washington DC is better served than any other area because it is in essence only a city, and urban areas are generally better supplied with physicians than are rural areas. In addition, it is a city with three medical schools, each having a cadre of doctors on staff.

The other end of the spectrum of the availability of physicians is occupied by states in the South and Mountain West. These states have less than half as many physicians per capita as do the best-served states. There are several reasons for this difference. One is that these states are less affluent than those with more physicians, so locating there may be less attractive economically. Not only will income opportunities for physicians be less, but there will likely be less of the high-tech equipment available that enables them to practice at the state of the art. And medical professionals, like all workers in science and technology, tend to prefer to work where there is a concentration of those professionals.

The distribution of the number of hospital beds per capita is rather different from the distribution of physicians. Several states in the West and South have higher numbers of hospital beds per capita than do more affluent and urbanized states. This reflects in part the economies of scale. The states with high numbers of hospital beds per capita have relatively small and dispersed populations, and therefore providing any level of access across the territory of the state may require higher numbers of beds than might be efficient in other settings. But this does not mean, however, that these rural states are really well-served, as I will point out below.

There are "healthcare deserts" in the United States that deprive many citizens of ready access to care. These are areas, urban as well as rural, in which there is no ready access to medical care, and often not even to a pharmacy. If someone wants medical care, they must travel miles in order to get even to a PCP, much less to more specialized care. For example, in the state of Kentucky, which is not the most rural of the states, 14 of 120 counties have no hospital. Further, these healthcare deserts often coincide with "food deserts" in which there may be no food stores other than convenience stores that offer only processed foods.

The problem of healthcare deserts has been, if anything, increasing over the past several decades. This has been primarily the result of the closing of a number of small rural hospitals. Over 130 rural hospitals have closed since 2010, with 27 closing in 2020 and 2021 (American Hospital Association, 2022). These hospitals had been central features of the healthcare systems in rural communities, but they were closing before the pandemic hit, and the pandemic was the death knell for many of them. Many did not have the capacity to treat severe COVID-19 cases but, more importantly, they were prevented from doing the elective surgeries that were their major income stream. Likewise, smaller, dispersed medical facilities in urban areas also have been closing, meaning that emergency care for severe problems is likely to be farther away.

The effects of the loss of rural hospitals can be seen in Table 7.5.[5] These hospitals have depended on elective surgeries for much of their income, but with the pandemic potential patients postponed surgeries, fearing infection if they went to the hospital (Best et al., 2020).

The problems of rural hospitals were made potentially worse in 2023 when a new payment regime was introduced (Beard, 2023). This new form of payment gave the hospitals more money for emergency room care, but on the condition that they stop providing in-patient care. In-patient care was a source of revenue for the hospitals, and also meant that emergency room staff could work in the in-patient wards of the hospital when there were no emergency patients. For areas where local hospitals accept this plan, patients will have to be transported long distances for in-patient care.

It is not just access to doctors and hospitals that may be limited in some parts of the country. During the COVID-19 pandemic pharmacies were important for distributing the vaccine. Most Americans have a pharmacy a mile or two from their homes, but pharmacy deserts exist and may be becoming more common. In 111 counties, mostly between the Mississippi and the Rockies, there is no pharmacy,

Table 7.5: Effects of closing rural hospitals: average distance in miles to facility offering types of treatment

	General Inpatient	Emergency Department	Alcohol or Drug	Cardiac Unit
2012	3.4	3.3	5.5	4.6
2018	23.9	24.2	44.6	35.1

Source: USGAO (2020).

much less one with storage facilities that could provide the extreme cold storage needed for the Pfizer and Moderna vaccines (Ullrich and Mueller, 2021).

Questions of transportation must also be added to the problems of geography in access to healthcare. That factor is obvious in rural areas where individuals may have to drive many miles to reach even a physician, much less a hospital. Although almost all people living in rural areas will have a vehicle, there are still those who do not. And in cities more people will depend upon public transportation that may or may not be convenient for reaching providers, especially if the individual is coping with an illness at the time.

Some private sector firms have been stepping in to attempt to address some of these problems of access. A number of drug store companies, such as CVS and Walgrens, are beginning to have medical practitioners in their stores, or online, for walk-in patients (Hart, 2022). Online retail giant Amazon is also entering the healthcare field, attempting to purchase one or more "urgicare" providers and link them with the online services that Amazon have already proven to manage so effectively. What is less clear about these innovations is how they will interface with existing insurance schemes, and whether they will be able to maintain high quality care.

Age

As well as highlighting some of the geographical disparities in health access in the United States, the COVID-19 pandemic highlighted disparities by age. The somewhat chaotic distribution of the vaccine in many states required individuals wishing to receive the vaccine to go online to various sites to try to locate a source, or to make numerous phone calls to pharmacies. Many older citizens, who needed the vaccine most, were unable to navigate the technology involved and, unless they had assistance from younger or more computer-literate family or friends, were delayed in getting the shots. Nominally those over 75 were first in line, but in practice that priority was meaningless because of the technical problems.

This problem of computer literacy, as well as cognitive impairments, among the older segments of the population was especially evident in dealing with vaccinations. This may, however, be a continuing problem, at least until those cohorts who grew up using computers reach their senior years. The pandemic has caused a large increase in the use of telemedicine, which requires the ability to use a computer or other device, and perhaps also may require a different way of interacting than does a face-to-face encounter with a healthcare provider. If this is the future of medicine, as it appears to be, then there may be negative results for older and other less computer-literate patients.

In addition to the specific problems associated with the use of technology, older patients may experience a general "ageism" in communications with their healthcare providers (Adelman et al., 2000). This negative response to the elderly includes tendencies of physicians to trivialize complaints by older patients, spending less time with older patients, and being less willing to suggest preventative measures or treat complaints aggressively. Thus, even though older patients may be able to go to the doctor with their Medicare card, their treatment and their ability to communicate their needs and worries may be limited.

Communications for access

When we discuss access to healthcare we need to consider not only formal access but also "real" access available to citizens. That is, it is not sufficient just to be able to get in the door but, once meeting with doctors or other healthcare providers, the information and wishes of the patient must be taken seriously. There is a great deal of evidence that minority group members and women tend to have more difficulties in having their complaints taken seriously, even by female and Black or Latino/a doctors, and this makes their effective access to healthcare less than it might appear.

The same difficulties in communications may be associated with class and educational differences. Many healthcare professionals may attribute these difficulties to the inability of some patients to communicate effectively. Patients may attribute the difficulties to the capacity of the professionals to listen effectively, and to explain admittedly complex medical issues in more everyday language. These communication difficulties may also be seen as a problem of hierarchy, and even of stigmatization. On the one hand, patients may be unwilling to challenge the authority and status of medical professionals. On the other hand, there is evidence that low-income patients believe they are being stigmatized for their low income, and for using public insurance (Allen et al., 2014). These communication problems obviously create problems of effective access for some patients when they are interacting with medical professionals and, more importantly, perhaps these issues may deter them from even seeking medical care.

Systemic barriers to access

The economic barriers to access to healthcare in the United States are significant and, indeed, are so significant that it is easy to overlook all the other factors that can inhibit an individual from gaining access. One of the more important of the additional factors is the structure of the medical care system itself. As I argued in the introductory chapter, much of the character of American healthcare is defined by the roles of insurance companies and private providers. Despite the critiques by many conservatives, although government is a major funder of medical care it is less influential in shaping the institutions delivering the services.

Several structural aspects of the healthcare system are especially important for limiting easy access for patients. The first and perhaps most important is the relatively small, and declining, proportion of physicians involved in primary care. PCPs are the primary gatekeepers in the healthcare system. But, as demonstrated in Table 7.6, PCPs have been declining for decades as a percentage of total physicians.

Table 7.6: Changing distribution of specialties of physicians

	1980	1990	2000	2010	2019
General Practice	17.6	15.2	13.1	8.2	7.9
Obstetrics and Gynecology	7.2	7.0	6.4	5.9	5.4
Surgery	11.4	12.1	12.9	13.6	13.9
Internal Medicine	8.7	9.0	9.4	9.6	9.9

Source: Kaiser Family Foundation, *Professionally Active Physicians*, various years.

The principal problem with this declining number of PCPs is that they are the ones providing routine, and importantly preventive, care for patients. Some specialists in internal medicine also function as PCPs, but the growth in that specialty has not made up for the loss in general practitioners.

Under many health insurance programs, individuals who want to see a specialist have to be referred by their PCP if they want the visit to the specialist to be covered by insurance. This requirement, of course, keeps the patient within the same network of physicians associated with the health insurer, but also makes it that much harder for individuals to move easily within the "jungle" of the healthcare industry. Many people of limited means and without stable social connections may find it difficult to maintain a relationship with a PCP, and therefore will face more barriers to gaining access to higher quality care. Further, having a long-term relationship with a PCP tends to produce better care for the patient, given that the doctor knows the patient's history and has at hand all the records of past visits.

The relative dearth of PCPs is, in some instances, exacerbated by restrictions on the activities of alternative healthcare providers such as nurse practitioners and physician assistants. Many of the tasks performed by PCPs are routine, and could be handled by trained professionals with less education than an MD (Doctor of Medicine). Many states, however, restrict the activities of these professionals, which consumes the time available from the PCPs for more detailed services (AAPA, 2022), and also increases the costs of providing the services (Chapter 8). Using nurse practitioners and physician assistants to provide the equivalent of PCP services for many routine issues could thus improve access with less additional cost, or probably with cost savings.

As well as a relatively low number of PCPs in the United States, there is an even greater dearth of geriatricians. Although the American population continues to become older, very few doctors with a specialty in geriatric medicine are in practice.[6] This small number of geriatricians is not simply a question of labeling. Most people think that surely a PCP can handle the medical needs of the elderly as well as those of other adults. But this can have real consequences for the health of the elderly (Sedhom and Barile, 2017). Many diseases present differently in older patients, and the communication problems between doctor and patient may also be exacerbated by cognitive loss.

Although the number of PCPs and geriatricians is especially important for providing access for patients, given that they are the gatekeepers of the medical care system, the overall number of physicians in the United States does not facilitate access, and also may increase costs because of reduced supply (see Chapter 8). The United States has relatively fewer doctors per capita than do many other wealthy countries. The number of MDs being produced by medical schools has increased (Boyle, 2021), but the number of new doctors has not kept pace with the increase in population and, despite the influx of a number of foreign medical graduates, the number of doctors in the United States remains relatively low relative to the population. Partly, the low number of doctors is a function of actions by several hierarchical actors. The medical profession itself controls supply, but the federal government is also responsible because of underfunding residency positions, so graduates of medical schools may not be able to find places to complete their training (Wofford, 2020).

The relatively small number of hospital beds in the United States is another possible barrier to access. During normal times this is not a real problem, given that many surgeries and other treatments that once required hospitalization are now done on an outpatient basis, in "same-day" surgery centers within hospitals, or managed independently from hospitals. The model of surgery has been promoted by the insurance companies as a means of reducing costs, and in general the outcomes of these surgeries are as good as the same procedure involving hospital care.[7] Although one sees massive hospital buildings scattered through cities, and even in some rural areas, the United States has fewer hospital beds per capita than many other industrialized countries (Table 7.7), representing the declining power of hospitals relative to insurance companies in the politics of healthcare, as well as more general shifts in patterns of medical care toward ambulatory care.

In addition to the structural barriers to access, some of the other factors mentioned above for individual access may also affect access systemically. For example, the comparative evidence is that, although the differences are small, the level of communication between doctors and patients in the United States is not as effective as in many other consolidated democracies (see Table 7.8). There may be any number of reasons for this deficiency, but the time pressures faced by physicians in the United States (Konrad et al., 2010) remain a source of "burnout" for physicians, as well as of the perception of the doctor being rushed while with patients.

How to improve access? Challenges for the future

There have certainly been improvements in the access of Americans to healthcare over the past several decades, but there are still a number of significant problems. While the ACA made it feasible for many more people to purchase insurance, with the expansion of Medicaid providing insurance to millions more who could not purchase it, there are still millions without insurance. Further, the number

Table 7.7: Hospital beds (per 1,000 population)

Germany	8.0
Austria	7.3
Poland	6.5
France	5.9
Belgium	5.6
Switzerland	4.6
Slovenia	4.4
Netherlands	3.2
United States	2.9
Canada	2.5
United Kingdom	2.5
Sweden	2.1

Source: World Bank, https://data.worldbank.org/indicator/SH.MED.BEDS.ZS.

Table 7.8: Patient satisfaction with interactions with physicians (2016, in percentage)

	Clear Communications	Shared Decision-making
Netherlands	96.9	87.1
Australia	93.5	87.9
Switzerland	90.7	86.5
United Kingdom	90.6	88.9
United States	89.5	84.6
Canada	88.0	84.3
Germany	85.9	87.6
France	83.7	78.8
Sweden	—	79.0
Average	89.2	85.0

Source: Kaiser Family Foundation, *Health System Tracker*, https://www.healthsystemtracker.org/indicator/access-affordability/communication-with-providers/.

without insurance increased during the pandemic, as people losing jobs also lost insurance and others chose not to continue insurance purchased through the ACA.

As well as the improvements in access that depend on improving access to insurance for individuals, there are systemic remedies that would improve access significantly. Perhaps the most important of these reforms would be to improve the availability of services in rural areas.

In addition to improving access in rural areas, improving access in poorly served areas within cities and suburbs would also enhance healthcare. These healthcare deserts are primarily in areas with high levels of poverty and minority populations without insurance. In economic terms this means that there is less demand for services, although almost certainly more need, and hence providers may choose not to locate there. Some of the same mechanisms that could be used for expanding services in rural areas could also be used to expand services in these other poorly served areas.

Some programs already exist that attempt to improve the distribution of healthcare facilities. For example, Medicare and Medicaid pay a 10 percent bonus for services provided by rural hospitals or facilities operating in underserved parts of the country. State governments that have large rural areas have also developed programs to get medical care to remote communities. These include having doctors and nurses available by air, and training local residents to handle low-level medical problems for other citizens.[8] However, as rural populations continue to decline, there will be even greater challenges in making modern medical care available in a timely and cost-effective manner.

Given that the number of physicians remaining in active practice is declining, there is another serious problem for access emerging. The "burnout" rate for physicians has been increasing, and did so dramatically during the pandemic (Greep et al., 2021). Much of the burnout of physicians is attributed to the administrative parts of their jobs—their need to fight through the jungle of insurers and regulators—rather than to the actual practice of medicine with patients (Patel et al., 2018). Coping with insurance company forms and procedures, and the increasing numbers of quality surveys and systems, takes time away from the things that motivated most medical practitioners to get into that profession. Even residents still in training are now experiencing burnout (AMA, 2022) and may not finish their training. Nurses are also leaving their jobs in droves after the pandemic (Mensik, 2022). They were hailed as heroes during the crisis, but now find that their workloads are unsustainable over longer periods.

The biggest challenge to access to healthcare will almost certainly remain financial. Despite the ACA, millions of people are uninsured or underinsured, and therefore do not have the ease of access that most Americans now have. And even for those who are insured the amount of money that now must be paid out of pocket to use the insurance can pose a significant barrier to access. These continuing financial barriers help motivate the continuing struggle to create a more truly universal health insurance system in the United States. That struggle to expand access will be discussed in Chapter 10.

8

Healthcare costs and cost containment

The second major issue in health policy is cost. American healthcare is expensive, and the United States devotes a larger share of its economic resources to health than do other advanced democracies. When the higher gross national product of the United States is considered, the differences in healthcare spending between the United States and the rest of the world is even more pronounced. As of 2022, healthcare accounts for over 17 percent of total economic activity This chapter will discuss why there is such a disproportionate level of spending for healthcare in the United States, and some of the options for controlling increases in cost.

One way of understanding the increasing costs of healthcare in the United States is to look at the increase in prices for healthcare relative to the rest of the economy. Medical price inflation, as can be seen from Table 8.1, has been proceeding much more rapidly than price inflation in other sectors of the economy. In most years the price increases for total medical services—meaning doctors and hospitals as well as other services—are at least double those of the total consumer price index.[1] There was some slight decrease in medical price inflation toward the end of the period covered by this table, in part a function of the COVID-19 pandemic, but the relative costs of healthcare continue to grow.

The rate of price increases for prescription drugs was not as great as might have been expected given the political pressures to control these costs (see pp. 128–32). Some of the political pressure has been created by extreme increases for some particular medications—notably insulin for diabetes—that affect some people extremely badly (Cohen, 2021). At the same time, however, more drugs have been moving off patent and are available as generics, reducing the total rate of increase of drug prices.

A similar measure of the cost of healthcare in the United States is the amount of money that the average family spends on healthcare. Table 8.2 shows that spending from 2012 to 2022. This table highlights two things about the costs of healthcare. The first is that the average family spends a great deal of money for healthcare. In 2022 the average family is spending over one-quarter of their median household income on healthcare. This is true even after the increasing involvement of government in healthcare, for example the Affordable Care Act. American families spend a great deal of money out of pocket for healthcare. This is true even if the family has health insurance, because the high, and increasingly higher, premiums, co-payments and deductibles charged have shifted more of the costs onto individuals and families.

Table 8.2 shows the average spending by families, but what it does not show is the amount of spending that an individual or family may make when they are faced with a major illness or accident. Even after the passage of the Affordable Care Act medical debt in the United States is massive, and is one of the leading

Table 8.1: Health cost inflation rates (annual price increases, in percentage)

	Total CPI[1]	Hospital Health	Prescription Services	Drugs
2012	2.1	3.2	5.1	3.6
2013	1.5	2.0	4.7	3.4
2014	1.6	3.0	5.0	3.6
2015	0.1	2.6	4.1	4.8
2016	1.3	4.1	4.5	3.4
2017	2.1	1.8	4.9	4.6
2018	2.4	2.0	4.4	1.6
2019	1.8	4.5	2.0	1.5
2020	1.2	1.8	4.2	1.0
2021	4.7	2.2	3.0	−1.8

[1] Consumer Price Index—general measure of all prices for consumers.
Source: US Department of Labor, Bureau of Labor Statistics, https://www.bls.gov/cpi/factsheets/medical-care.htm.

Table 8.2: Estimated out-of-pocket spending for medical care for a family of four (in dollars)

2022	30,260
2021	28,256
2020	26,078
2019	27,233
2018	28,166
2017	26,944
2016	25,826
2015	24,671
2014	23,215
2013	22,030
2012	22,079

Source: *Milliman Medical Index*, annual.

causes of personal bankruptcy (Himmelstein et al., 2019; Carroll, 2022). Insurance policies may have caps on total expenditures per person, but those caps can easily be exceeded by a major illness or injury, especially if it involves long-term nursing care. It is also important to remember that it is not just individuals who are paying soaring healthcare costs. Businesses that provide insurance for their workers are also facing very high and increasing costs (Altman, 2021).

The impact of serious disease on personal finances can be seen in Table 8.3 that compares the financial situations and behaviors of patients who have been treated for cancer. Almost two-thirds of respondents who have been treated for cancer say

Table 8.3: Impact of cancer incident on personal finances (by percentage)

	Cancer Diagnosis	No Cancer
Used up Most of Savings	60	46
Declared Bankruptcy or Lost Home	23	16
Withdrew Money from College or Retirement Savings	43	27
Changed Living Situation, e.g. Moved in with Family	29	17
Skipped or Delayed Medical Treatments	74	67

Source: Levey (2022).

they have exhausted their savings in the process, as compared to just over a quarter of non-cancer patients who also reported financial troubles from healthcare. Other variables do not show as much impact from an incident of cancer. But the basic point remains that even being insured does not protect patients against financial crises from serious illnesses or accidents.

The other thing that Table 8.2 demonstrates, as does Table 8.1, is that the healthcare costs continue to increase. These costs have increased in real terms as well as in nominal terms, and as a percentage of median family income. Healthcare is becoming a more significant expense for the average family. Thus, total spending on healthcare as a percentage of gross domestic product continues to increase, and the amount of spending by ordinary citizens also continues to increase. There was a slight decrease in 2020 and in 2021 because people had fewer surgeries and fewer doctors' visits during the pandemic, but rates of spending on healthcare are increasing rapidly in 2022 as people begin to have treatments that were postponed during the pandemic.

Why does healthcare cost so much in the United States?

In all healthcare systems there are a number of factors that make controlling costs more difficult than in other parts of the economy, or other policy domains. These factors may be especially powerful in the United States, but they are present everywhere and present difficulties for political and administrative leaders. As I will point out below, many of the pressures on healthcare and the associated costs are likely to continue to increase, and again those pressures are likely to be especially powerful in the United States. Given that, the second part of this chapter will focus on possible means of controlling costs.

The first driver of costs is simply that healthcare involves professional services, high levels of technology, medications involving substantial research and testing, and often an extensive amount of time for hospitalization and for continuing treatments. Any service that has those characteristics will cost a great deal, and any modern healthcare system will be expensive. And it is a service that everybody needs and wants, so demand drives up costs. This is, of course, especially true in fee-for-service medicine such as in the United States, but it is also a factor in healthcare systems that operate without separate payments for each service or product.

The fee–for–service nature of healthcare pricing in the United States makes the underlying pressure from costs of professional services even greater. Most Americans incur a separate bill every time they see their doctor, every time they have a blood test, and every time they receive any other tests or treatments. This basis for charging the patients gives the medical providers few incentives to be economical with services, and indeed the pressures are in the direction of providing more services, and hence creating higher total costs. That said, the incentives for the insurance companies are to restrict the amount of service and thereby to increase their profits.

A second and closely related common driver of healthcare costs is that there are powerful actors involved, and those actors may be able to evade controls that are imposed on other parts of the economy. In most societies medical professionals are viewed with respect, or even awe, and may be able to elude cost controls placed on other actors. Likewise, institutions such as hospitals are major employers, and in local settings may be too powerful to control effectively. Even when the health sector is dominated by government, popular support for good healthcare may prevent clamping down on spending and endangering quality. The National Health Service (NHS) in the United Kingdom is one of the more tightly controlled health systems in a democratic country, but political leaders or managers who want to constrain costs still encounter major problems (Klein, 2019; Abbasi, 2020), and there is political capital to be made by arguing for more money for the NHS.

The employees of healthcare systems are not just doctors and nurses. There is a much larger number of technicians, orderlies, cleaners and food service workers who are employed in the health sector. Not only are these employees important in local economies, they are often unionized—as are doctors and nurses in many settings—and can wield this organizational power to maintain or increase their wages. No political leader, or healthcare executive, wants to be faced with the scene of healthcare workers picketing hospitals and preventing needed care for patients.

Like all healthcare workers, those unionized workers are feeling "burnout" after the pandemic, and are pressing demands for high salaries and better working conditions that will contribute to higher expenditures.

In addition to economic and political power exercised by healthcare providers, demand from the public for healthcare seems virtually insatiable. People want to feel better, be more active and see medical care as one major means of achieving those goals. Thus, especially when the health system is controlled by government, the public will exert pressure to maintain and expand healthcare. Even in the (somewhat) market-based medical system of the United States politicians who want to tamper with existing health programs encounter strong opposition.[2] Medicare, in particular, has become a "third rail" of American politics, along with social security, that no ambitious politician wants to touch.

There are pressures from both the supply side and demand side for increased spending on healthcare. There are some more issues in service delivery that tend to make controlling costs difficult. One standard means of reducing spending in any field is to reduce waste. Some estimates of waste are that it is almost a third of spending on healthcare, but even more conservative estimates are that billions of dollars are lost each year through waste of various types.

But defining waste in healthcare can be more difficult (see Shrank et al., 2019). For example, someone may say that ordering a number of tests on a patient with vague symptoms is wasteful, but it is not so wasteful if the tests reveal a serious underlying disease. Indeed, one of the common concerns of minority and publicly insured patients is that they do not receive adequate testing and therefore diseases are not detected until they have become more severe. Likewise, some people may consider the prices they are charging as perfectly reasonable, while others may consider them extortionate and excessive.

Medical care is a very different market or service than most others. It is difficult to know in advance what the quality of the "product" will be. Patients may know by reputation which hospitals or doctors are supposed to be the best, but even then there may be less information than when buying a new car or mobile phone. Given this lack of information, patients may opt for the highest priced service as a surrogate indicator for quality. Even when there is a dominant public role in healthcare, patients can opt for private medical care, again assuming that the quality will be higher. These choices, based on inadequate information, will tend to drive up total healthcare spending and do so perhaps unnecessarily.

And finally, almost all countries in the world are being faced with severe demographic pressures on health spending. Spending on medical care tends to increase as an individual passes the mid-50s, and tends to increase more rapidly in the individuals' 70s and 80s. As Tables 8.4 and 8.5 show, health spending for over 65s is higher than in other age groups, and individuals over 85—sometimes referred to as the "old-old"—consume a disproportionate share of health spending. Because the medical care systems in industrial countries have been successful in helping more of their population to live much longer, they have created increasing pressures on health spending. Further, given declining birth rates and the generally

Table 8.4: Age and healthcare spending, 2019

Age	Percentage of Population	Percentage of Health Spending
0–18	24	9
19–34	21	12
35–44	13	9
45–54	13	13
55–64	13	21
65+	17	35

Source: Kaiser Family Foundation, *Health Tracker*, November 12, 2021.

Table 8.5: Age and Medicare spending (known)

Age	Percentage of Enrolled	Percentage of Spending
Under 65	16.7	17.3
65–74	42.2	32.2
74–85	26.3	31.3
85+	12.7	16.2

Source: Center for Medicare and Medicaid Studies (2022).

increasing longevity, the financial and service pressures on the health system will continue to increase.

Drivers of cost in American healthcare

In addition to the general drivers of costs in healthcare, there are some drivers that are more specific to the United States, and its more widespread use of the private sector—for both insurance and providers—than is true for other countries. The absence of central government controls over health spending and the power of private actors such as drug companies means that there are few effective controls over spending. Health insurance companies are the major actors with a direct interest in containing costs, but even they have not been able to restrain spending. This is in part because of the trade-off between quality and cost. Patients demand newer treatments and newer drugs, as do their doctors, and those purchases are driving up the total cost of healthcare.

Perhaps the most fundamental cause for the high costs of medical care in the United States is fee-for-service medicine. As already discussed, most health services are charged as they are delivered, whether they are part of a network or not. The major exception is the relatively high number of Americans belonging to health maintenance organizations (HMOs) (approximately 32 percent). While this system of payment is similar to other commercial transactions, it does give a provider an incentive to provide more services than might really be necessary. This appears to occur especially for people with good insurance who will not themselves bear most of the cost, so it may be perceived as relatively costless—except, of course, the insurance company is paying, and those costs are passed on as higher premiums.

Fragmentation

The fragmentation of the healthcare system in the United States, which some analysts tend to regard as a virtue because it can be related to higher levels of competition, is a fundamental structural factor in higher costs. This fragmentation is one aspect of the jungle that exists in medical care, as outlined in Chapter 1. In addition to the effects of competition (see below) fragmentation is associated with inefficiencies, duplication and inadequate coordination. For patients, the fragmentation also increases the complexity of the healthcare system, which in turn creates confusion, and may negatively affect access as well as increase overall costs within the system.

Fragmentation can be managed, but there are few coordinating devices within the American healthcare system. In principle the primary care physician (PCP) should be coordinating care for their patients, but that can be a daunting task. Coordinating care requires dealing with a number of actors that may not want to be coordinated, and in the case of specialists, may have higher status in the medical world than the PCP. Insurance companies also attempt to coordinate care, albeit primarily to protect their own economic interests rather than to provide better services to patients. Further, patients themselves may resist coordination, especially as they may be able to contact specialists without referrals, and may pursue treatment from several different PCPs if they have the economic resources.

The fee-for-service nature of American medicine also creates incentives for actors to seek profits through fragmenting services. HMOs have been used as a remedy for fragmentation and the effects of fee-for-service medicine since the 1970s. The Health Maintenance Organization Act of 1973 requires employers with over 25 employees to offer an HMO if they provide other forms of health coverage (Falkson and Srinivasan, 2022). Despite that, HMOs cover only about one-third of the population. Given that HMOs charge a single fee for all services for a time period, they have no incentive to provide additional services. Indeed, the problem with this form of medical care organization may be that they have an incentive not to provide services, including some testing that could catch conditions early.

Price intransparency

When a consumer goes into a shop to buy most products, they will soon know what the price is. This openness about price is rarely true for medical care, other than knowing what the co-pay associated with their insurance policy may be. If the "customer" does have insurance they may not care about the total cost. Further, the quote that is made for the cost of surgery or other procedures may only be an estimate, given the variable costs that may be added during a hospital stay. If the patient has complications, or needs any special treatment, then the cost of the hospital stay will escalate.

The federal government has enacted regulations that require providers to post their prices for a number of services that they provide (Furlow, 2019). The Affordable Care Act contained the first requirements of this sort, and those requirements were extended during the Trump administration. As providers— especially hospitals—begin to implement these rules, however, the results have been disappointing (Kurani et al., 2021a). One problem is that the same service may cost different amounts even within the same hospital, depending upon agreements between insurers and the hospital. For example, prices for a lower spine MRI in one Idaho hospital ranged from under $1,000 to almost $5,000.

In addition, less than 10 percent of the American population are aware of the requirements for providers to give patients price information (Kurani et al., 2021b). Although there are requirements to reveal prices, providers have been slow to comply (Kack, 2023).

Emergency care has become one of the major areas of intransparency in pricing for patients. When someone has a medical emergency they rarely think about all the cost implications, and these can be significant. Although Congress has passed a "No Surprises" bill for emergency services, there are still numerous cases in which privately insured patients will pay out-of-network bills for services such as ambulance rides that will run into the thousands of dollars (Amin et al., 2021). And at the emergency rooms they may be charged a "trauma team activation fee" even if there is no serious trauma (Gold and Kliff, 2018).

Administration

The competitive nature of healthcare in the United States, whether it works or not to reduce some costs, also imposes other costs. That competition, and the associated fragmentation of the system, produce administrative costs in the US health system that are substantially higher than in other countries. These administrative costs appear in many aspects of healthcare, but appear most clearly in the insurance system and in hospitals. Further, given that much of the medical care system is in the private or the not-for-profit sectors, the salaries being paid to many people managing healthcare companies and facilities are often extremely high.

The administrative costs arising from insurance in the United States are much higher in the private sector than in the public sector (Himmelstein et al., 2020). The administrative costs for the United States tend to be at least double those of other OECD countries as a percentage of current spending on health. The countries that are closest to the United States—Germany, Austria and Switzerland—tend also to be countries that are higher spenders than are the other countries. It appears that higher spending for administration is a significant contributing factor to higher levels of total spending.

Despite the usual claims of efficiency in the private sector, the administrative costs in the United States are especially high for private insurance, and for Medicare Part C, which is managed by private sector firms (Table 8.6). Taken together, the administrative expenses for insurers in the United States as a percentage of total expenditures are 2.5 times greater than those in Canada, although the administrative expenses of US private insurers are slightly less than those of private insurers in Canada. The same is generally true for the administrative costs of providers, which are much higher in the United States than in Canada.

The high costs of administration in the United States is explained by a number of factors. One which is often cited is the large number of employees involved in coding claims from different insurance companies that use different systems. One standard remedy for high costs, therefore, is to have one form for all insurance, along with one set of codes to classify diagnoses and treatments.

Table 8.6: Administrative costs as a percentage of total health expenditure, 2017

United States	8.3
France	5.7
Germany	4.2
Netherlands	3.9
Switzerland	3.8
Australia	3.0
Canada	2.7
Denmark	2.4
United Kingdom	2.0
Japan	1.6
Sweden	1.4

Source: OECD, *Health Care Expenditures and Finances*, 2019.

A single-payer insurance system (see Chapter 10) would be the simplest solution administratively, but would encounter a number of political hurdles. Creating a common form through regulations would, however, go a long way to solving the problem.

Another reason for the extremely high administrative costs in American healthcare is the high salaries paid to executives in the private firms, especially those in health insurance. These firms are competing with other corporations in the private market for executive talent, while most public employees are paid on a fixed pay scale.[3] Table 8.7 provides information on some of the higher paid chief executive officers (CEOs) in healthcare organizations, although it leaves out the salaries of CEOs of pharmaceutical firms.

Advertising is another aspect of overhead costs that affects the private sector dominated health system in the United States. Given that health insurance companies and hospitals are in competition with one another, they engage in all the activities that private sector organizations do in order to improve their market position. The level of spending is not easy to calculate, but it was roughly $10 billion in 2017, and was expected to increase to $11.6 billion by 2021 (Minemyer, 2018).

Technology

The development of technology represents another important driver of costs in American health policy. Modern medical technology can do wonders in diagnosing health problems and in delivering cures. The advances in imaging technology and in extremely precise radiation for treating cancer are but two rather obvious examples. But these advances in medical technology come at a price. A new MRI machine can easily cost $3 million, plus setting up the space to house it, and hiring

Table 8.7: Highest paid executives in healthcare, 2020 (in dollars; excluding pharmaceuticals)

Michael Neidorff (Centene)	25 million
David M. Cordani (Cigna)	19.8 million
Samuel Hazen (HCA)	18.1 million
Joseph Zubretsky (Molina Healthcare)	17.8 million
Bruce Broussard (Humana)	16.5 million
Michael Kaufmann (Cardinal Health)	14.2 million

Source: Equilar Insight, https://www.equilar.com/reports/80-highest-paid-ceos-2021-equilar-100.html.

Table 8.8: MRIs (per one million inhabitants, 2019)

Japan	55.2
United States	40.4
Germany	34.7
Austria	23.5
Comparable Country Average	22.3
France	15.4
Australia	14.8
Netherlands	13.1
Belgium	11.6
Canada	10.4

Source: Kaiser Family Foundation, *Health System Tracker*, https://www.healthsystemtracker.org/chart-col lection/u-s-health-care-resources-compare-countries/#Nurses%20licensed%20to%20practice,%20dens ity%20per%201,000%20population,%202000-2018.

the technicians to run it. Depending on a number of factors, the base price for a MRI scan will be between $1,000 and $4,000 (GE Healthcare, 2019).

Technology is a factor in driving costs in the United States in part because we use so much of it. In 2019 the United States had approximately twice as many MRI scanners per capita as other comparable countries (see Table 8.8). Hospitals compete to have the best doctors on their staffs,[4] and therefore need to have all the best equipment available to attract and retain those doctors. Likewise, patients like to be able to get these imaging services as close to home as they can. The proliferation of MRIs and other imaging technologies may be positive in some ways, especially if one is attempting to argue that US healthcare is the best in the world, but it does add to the total costs of healthcare.

Certificates of need are used in some states to control the purchase of technology, as well as hospitals and other medical facilities. As of 2022 35 states have certificate of need laws, or have a moratorium of certain types of medical facilities or activities (NCSL, 2022). Under these laws, a healthcare provider must demonstrate a need for the investment in new facilities or services. These laws were originally mandated by the federal government but, while federal controls have largely expired, many states continue to use these laws for health planning and to control costs.

The purchase of the diagnostic machinery will impose significant capital costs on the facility that purchases it. That cost must be recovered through multiple uses, and there are some concerns that the scanning machinery is over-used. The over-use is argued to be especially likely for proprietary organizations that may have a profit motive (Span, 2022). This in turn leads also to a question of quality if patients are receiving unnecessary testing and perhaps treatment (see Chapter 9).

Drug costs

The final important driver of healthcare costs is the high price Americans pay for pharmaceuticals compared to the rest of the world. Although many of the major producers and developers of drugs are located in the United States, the same products cost much less in other countries (see Table 8.9). This disparity in costs is in part because Medicare has not used its market power to negotiate with drug companies, and indeed has been forbidden by law from doing so. The Inflation Reduction Act of 2022 has begun to change that, but initially only for ten drugs, and the fiscal year 2024 budget calls for expanding that negotiating power (Reed, 2023a). Some state governments do negotiate for better prices for bulk purchases, but the drug lobby has been sufficiently powerful to maintain its pricing advantages. Health insurance companies also try to control prices by having their own formularies of drugs that physicians in their networks can prescribe, but that mechanism appears relatively ineffective (Moore and Newman, 1993).[5]

These high prices of pharmaceuticals are vexing to American health consumers for several reasons. The first is that drugs are indeed expensive, and the coverage for drugs may be sporadic in health insurance plans. Even for people with health insurance, pharmaceuticals can be a major out-of-pocket expenditure. In addition,

Table 8.9: Drug prices compared: US drug prices as a percentage of prices in other countries

	Branded Originated Drugs	Generic Drugs
Canada	294	57
France	349	58
Germany	280	62
Italy	315	59
Japan	307	43
Mexico	367	56
United Kingdom	349	68
All Countries[1]	344	84

[1] OECD countries.

Source: Mulcahy et al. (2021).

the costs of drugs continue to increase, and in some cases do so dramatically. For example, the price of the EpiPen, a device that delivers a dose of epinephrine,[6] rose from $100 to $600 for two injectors, beginning in 2009 (Lyon, 2016). This increase was an especially egregious example that resulted from the rights being sold to a different firm that capitalized on the (then) monopoly, but similar examples do exist.

The second factor that irritates many Americans about drug prices is that they pay much higher prices for drugs than do consumers in other countries. For example, a report by the Rand Corporation (Mulcahy et al., 2021) found that Americans pay on average over 2.5 times as much for name-brand prescription drugs as do consumers in other similar countries. The differences for the 60 most frequently prescribed drugs is even greater—almost 400 percent—and the prices for drugs that originated in the United States are not substantially lower than the prices for all drugs (see Kurani et al., 2022).

The figures contained in Table 8.9 demonstrate yet a third irritating factor about American drug prices. Drug companies in the United States, and the American government, invest huge amounts of money in developing new pharmaceuticals, but that investment appears to benefit non-Americans as much or more than it does Americans. Drugs manufactured in the United States and shipped across the Atlantic are still cheaper there than in the cities in which they were manufactured. To many Americans this appears to be a significant error in policy, and an injustice.

Despite all the complaints that are being made about the prices of drugs, they are likely to increase. Even if there are reductions, or at least controls, on widely-used drugs, new drugs that are being developed may have astronomical prices. This is in part because drugs are being tailored to individual genetic characteristics. Medicines, especially for treating cancer, will be individualized and may cost in the hundreds of thousands or even millions of dollars per treatment. Few individuals will be able to afford those prices, and insurance companies may be very reluctant to authorize them.

Leaving aside the costs of drugs tailored to individuals, there are still very high-cost drugs entering the market that are likely to continue to put cost pressures on insurers. For example, in June, 2021 the Food and Drug Administration approved a new drug for Alzheimer's disease. This drug will cost an estimated $56,000 per year per patient, and is of special concern for Medicare given that most Alzheimer's patients are over 65 years of age (Bagley and Sachs, 2021). Given that this medication has to be given in a doctor's office, it is covered fully under Part B of Medicare, without any additional co-payments by the patient. The impact on Medicare's budget could have been catastrophic, but the medicine was later recalled for being ineffective.

At the time of writing, the federal government has done little to use its purchasing power, never mind its regulatory power, to control the price of drugs. Even though Medicare pays for billions of dollars of drugs it is only beginning to use that purchasing power to bargain for lower prices. Some of the states have created their own formularies and have bargained for lower drug prices for

Medicaid patients and for patients in state hospitals and prisons. States are also increasingly using managed care organizations to control spending on drugs, along with using more generic drugs (Dranove et al., 2017). And even when managed care is not utilized, the states purchase drugs in bulk.

The political power of "Big Pharma" is one of the major factors that maintains the high prices of pharmaceuticals in the United States (Sekerka and Benishek, 2018). The pharmaceutical industry is actually the largest single lobbyist in Washington, spending substantially more than the second-ranked industry (Frankenfield, 2020). This huge investment in lobbying has paid off in the unwillingness of government to impose any strong controls over the prices charged to citizens, and to government itself. President Biden's "Build Back Better" plan involved strong controls over drug prices, but a combination of lobbying by the drug companies and by citizens concerned about the loss of new, more effective drugs (especially for cancer) made passage difficult (Sanger-Katz, 2022).

Controlling costs: another philosopher's stone?

We know that healthcare services consume much more money than in other wealthy countries, and it would be logical to attempt to control those expenditures. This control of costs would benefit individual citizens, the employers who provide much of the health insurance for those citizens, and government. The question is why cost controls are not more effective, and why more effort is not exerted attempting to hold down the costs of healthcare. This is especially true given the power of health insurers—perhaps the clearest source of hierarchical power in the system—and their interest in controlling costs.

Competition

One commonly cited solution for rising costs in healthcare is more competition. This is a standard assumption in economics, with the logic being that competing producers will attempt to provide the product in question at the lowest possible price, and therefore will drive prices down. This argument has been advanced any number of times by Republicans and by conservative think tanks, and is especially prominent when the idea of a "single-payer" health plan (government being the single-payer) is advanced. The consolidation of resources in the single-payer plan is assumed by conservatives to make cost increases more likely since competition will be eliminated.

While this option has a great deal of credibility for many Americans, there are some important questions to be answered. The first is why is competition not working already? In my own area I have the option of a dozen or more health insurance companies, each with multiple plans. And there are three major healthcare networks, and numerous independent providers, all of which act like they are in a marketplace, for example they advertise extensively and try to corner their own share of the market. But even with all that competition prices continue to rise.

In fairness it should be noted that, living in an urban area, the density of providers of medical care and insurance is much greater than in some parts of the country. As noted in Chapter 7, for many Americans the question is not which hospital but rather whether there is any hospital at all. The same is true for health insurance, and in a few states there may be only a single option available for policies under the Affordable Care Act. So, some simple policy changes such as allowing competition by insurance companies across state lines may help create more of a marketplace in healthcare.

Arguably, one of the major reasons that competition does not work for healthcare is that providers want to create monopolies rather than to live with competition. In many major medical "marketplaces" there have been battles among insurers attempting to gain dominance, and hospitals also have been engaged in anti-competitive actions trying to enlarge their market shares and eliminate competition (Postma and Roos, 2015). In response to these anti-competitive behaviors, the Biden administration issued an extensive executive order to attempt to create more competition (Haefner, 2021). This order included rules such as slowing hospital mergers, promoting price transparency, and forbidding non-compete clauses for hiring healthcare personnel.

But the principal question is whether competition can work, and whether healthcare is just another commodity to be provided through the market (see Box 8.1). Some economists have argued that it is not such a commodity, and therefore competition is not a suitable remedy for cost increases, or for other problems within this sector (see Mankiw, 2017). Perhaps the dominant problem in a marketplace for health is that consumers do not know what they need, and what it is worth. Consumers know they want a new car, but may not know if they want (or need) medical procedures or pharmaceuticals. Hence, unlike other segments of the market, decisions are controlled by providers.

Box 8.1: Why health does not fit the market model

(1) The consumer cannot know a priori about the quality of the product.
(2) The producer, for example the medical profession, has excessive influence over the consumer.
(3) Entry of alternative providers into the market is limited.
(4) Consumption may not be voluntary, that is, if the patient becomes ill they must consume medical care.
(5) Competition may raise prices rather than lowering them.
(6) Consumers have little choice—they must use the providers offered to them by their insurance.
(7) There are few economies of scale—larger often means more expensive.

Derived, in part, from Rosenthal (2017).

In addition, competition may lead consumers to over-consume healthcare. Most of us are content with one car, or maybe two, but the demand for healthcare may be insatiable. If not insatiable then certainly people who have good insurance are likely to spend a great deal of insurance money on healthcare—more than they would if all the costs came directly out of pocket. Features of health insurance such as co-pays and deductibles may slow that consumption, but it is still higher than might be justified on economic or even health terms.

Competition may also increase rather than decrease spending. For example, hospitals may want to compete to have the best doctors practice in their facilities. Doing that will require investing in expensive equipment that then will have to be amortized across the bills for all patients. Similarly, health insurance companies spend billions of dollars on advertising each year to compete with one another ($23 billion in 2019; see also Schwartz and Wolshin, 2019), and those costs are reflected in the premiums that policyholders have to pay. Likewise, pharmaceutical companies spend billions in marketing drugs directly to consumers, as well as to medical professionals.[7] And, finally, the CEOs of major health firms and pharmaceutical firms expect to be paid like the CEOs of other major corporations, rather than being paid like a civil servant or a government minister.[8]

Value-based medical practice

Medical insurance programs, including public medical insurance programs such as Medicare, attempt to control the types of procedures that are unnecessary or unproven. But even then it appears that a large amount of money is being spent on procedures and pharmaceuticals that have little value, at least relative to their costs.

The principal question in value-based medicine—whether for reimbursements or for pricing—is whether the new or alternative technology is sufficiently superior to the established standard of care to justify additional expenditures. This question can be expressed in an equation[9] where ICER stands for "incremental cost efficiency ration" and QALY stands for "quality-adjusted life year". The assumption is if the ICER is above a certain threshold then the innovation is justified (Garrison and Towse, 2017).

There are several issues with applying this idea of value-based medicine. One issue is that any assessment of the utility of the innovation will necessarily be an average, but individuals may respond differently to different treatments, and perhaps especially different medications. Physicians and their staffs spend many hours arguing on behalf of their patients to have different medications approved by insurance companies, and the same types of arguments may have to be made for the innovative treatments. In the end, however, this may be a case in which averages may mask more than they reveal.

The second issue is how much should an increase in QALYs be worth? For an individual any improvement in their lifespan, and especially their lifespan with a high quality of life, may be worth a very great deal of money, but for society as a whole—and especially the funders of healthcare—that value must be weighed against alternative uses of the funds, both within healthcare and without. This disjuncture between individual demands and the total cost to society remains a challenge for health policymaking. An example of what may be excessive testing can help illustrate this point. One research study found that on average 1,000 women would have to undergo mammography for 11 years before one life could be saved from breast cancer (Keen and Keen, 2009).

Unfortunately for thinking about cost control, much of the evaluation of new technologies and procedures examines the effectiveness of individual interventions rather than their relative efficiency (Leonhardt, 2009). Many interventions that are effective may not be sufficiently valuable to displace other, lower cost forms of treatment, but the general cultural value in science and medicine appears to be that newer is better.

The COVID-19 pandemic has raised another important point about value in medical care. We generally think of value in terms of individuals who are receiving treatment. But if an individual is vaccinated they create values for many other people as well. Indeed, some of the marketing of vaccination to reluctant people has been that they are helping their neighbors and their country as a whole, not just themselves. For other types of medical interventions the value created for society is, however, less clear.

Controlling drug prices

The costs of pharmaceuticals are one of the major drivers of medical costs, and one that tends to irritate the average citizen perhaps more than others. For example, in one poll in 2021 (Kirzinger et al., 2021), reducing the costs of prescription drugs was the number one priority for improving healthcare among the respondents. This sense of priority is shared by employers who are paying high drug prices in their employee health insurance programs. That popular irritation about drug prices is accentuated because many drugs are developed in the United States, but are much cheaper elsewhere (Ess et al., 2003). The current high drug prices make it impossible for many patients to buy all the medications they need, or to take them on a regular basis. But despite the public discontent, drug prices have remained high, and have continued to increase.

The process by which drugs are manufactured and then eventually reach patients fits the jungle model discussed in Chapter 1 very well. Although there is a single regulator for the safety and efficacy of medications, the actual distribution depends on factors such as whether the drug is branded or is a generic, whether it is complex, compounded or a single molecule, and whether it is administered or dispensed (Waxman et al., 2020). For example, the prices for branded drugs in the United States are much higher than those in other countries, but generic medications tend to be lower.

Some of the suggestions for reducing prices are very simple. For example, many injectable drugs come in packages that contain more than one dose. This results in a great deal of waste, given that an individual physician may not have use of the remaining doses in the vial. Another simple proposal would be to promote greater transparency so that patients and their physicians would know what specific drugs would cost on insurance programs, and have the ability to take different pricing schemes into account (Feldman, 2022).

More extreme solutions are being introduced for the price of some drugs, notably insulin. Insulin prices have risen dramatically in the United States, costing many times what it costs in other countries: a vial of insulin that costs $21 in 1999 now costs over $300 (Rajkumar, 2020), with no apparent reason for the cost increases other than profits; it is a well-established drug involving little or no development costs. It is, however, produced by only a few companies that have exercised monopoly powers. In reaction, the state of California is undertaking manufacturing insulin for its Medicaid patients (Sherkow et al., 2023). Perhaps in response, manufacturers have begun to announce price reductions.

Using markets

One of the common recommendations for reducing the costs of drugs is to use the market power of Medicare and Medicaid to bargain with drug companies and intermediaries (pharmacy benefit managers), in much the same way that private insurers do. Medicare now has approximately 65 million people enrolled in the program. Approximately 40 percent of that number are in Medicare Advantage programs, some of which do provide lower rates on prescription drugs. Still, reducing spending on drugs by Medicare recipients would be doing so for a significant share of the population, and an even larger share of the prescription drugs, given that seniors tend to use many more drugs than other age groups.

Congress has specifically forbidden Medicare from negotiating with drug companies. This reflects the power of "Big Pharma" as one of the largest and most influential lobbyists in Washington. It is difficult to say just how much money could be saved by allowing negotiations, but it would be in the billions of dollars. One estimate in 2008 was that $21.9 billion could be saved if Medicare paid the same prices as other federal agencies, for example the Department of Veteran's Affairs (Gellad et al., 2008). A more recent study using prices from the Department estimated even larger savings (Frakt et al., 2011).

Another market-based solution for high drug prices would be to allow more drugs to be imported from Canada, or perhaps other countries as well. While it is illegal for individuals to import drugs for their personal use, beginning during the Trump administration the federal government has been developing means to assist the states in importing drugs, primarily for Medicaid. The Biden administration supported the rule proposed by Trump, and individual states can now seek waivers from the Department of Health and Human Services (HHS) to import. The Food and Drug Administration must approve the drugs being imported.[10]

The possibilities of reducing pharmaceutical costs through market power has been emphasized by Mark Cuban's Cost Plus Drug Company that sells generic drugs online for a 15 percent markup over the price from the manufacturer, plus a $3 dispensing fee and $5 shipping fee. A study reported in the *Annals of Internal Medicine* (Lalani et al., 2022) reported that Medicare could have saved over one-third of Part D's total expenditure had it used the plan developed by Cuban, a billionaire entrepreneur with a commitment to lowering medical costs. This plan is able to reduce prices by removing some of the "jungle" elements of dispensing pharmaceuticals, especially eliminating pharmacy benefit managers who operate as middlemen.[11] Critics of the Cuban program, however, argue that it only takes on the easy targets—generic drugs—rather than dealing with the much more expensive brand-name drugs (Twenter, 2022).

If market-based controls do not work, then direct regulation becomes the means to reduce the costs of prescription drugs. A number of different options for controlling drug prices have been proposed, all of which will require some direct intervention by government into the hierarchical system, controlled by the drug companies, that now determines prices. Those interventions may require some time to phase in, so that the drug manufacturers can adjust their ways of doing business over time, but in the end strong interventions from government may be required. That type of legislation will be difficult to pass, given attitudes of many Republican congressmen.[12]

Legislative proposals in the House of Representatives, called the Elijah E. Cummings Lower Drug Costs Now Act, would require the HHS to negotiate directly with drug companies on the prices of the 125 drugs that do not have a generic substitute available and that produce the most spending, either in total or for Medicare. The legislation requires HHS to negotiate prices that are either 120 percent of the average price in six industrial countries,[13] or 85 percent of the manufacturer price. Drug companies who choose not to participate would face civil fines and tax penalties. Also, private insurers that did not use the negotiated prices would be forbidden from insuring federal workers. A similar plan, confined initially to only ten pharmaceuticals, has been adopted by the Biden administration (Cubanski et al., 2023).

Another option for lowering drug prices would be to reform Medicare Part D. Part D is often characterized as a competitive program because there are multiple plans from which consumers can choose, based on price and coverage. However, much of the spending for Part D is hidden because of public sector "reinsurance" (Frakt et al., 2011). After the individual has reached a level on out-of-pocket payments (now $5,030) 80 percent of the costs of any more prescriptions are paid by government. This means that consumers assume their plan is working well for them, while in reality it is taxpayers who are paying for high drug prices.

One possible means of controlling drug costs could be to treat the pharmaceutical industry as a regulated utility, much as electricity and gas services are treated. These firms are guaranteed a return on capital but have their rates set so that they do not exceed the established rate of return. For drug companies this would mean that they could have a guaranteed return on their research and development expenses for drugs. This would require taking into account all the money that is spent researching drugs that never make it to market.

Table 8.10: Examples of state government actions to control drug prices (2017–2022, number of states adopting)

Regulating Pharmacy Benefit Managers	47
Importation	9
Price Transparency	21
Volume Purchasing	3
Affordability Reviews	8
Coupons/Cost-Sharing	22

Source: National Academy for State Health Policy, https://www.nashp.org/rx-laws/.

The discussion to this point has focused on controlling drug prices at the federal level, but the states have been active in this policy area (Gudiksen and King, 2019), and appear to be more successful in deflecting pressures from the pharmaceutical manufacturers. Although Medicaid is largely federally funded, it is administered by the states, and state governments have engaged in a number of programs to control drug costs (see Table 8.10). Some of these actions have been attacked in court by the drug companies, with limited success, but in most cases state governments have had the authority to implement these programs. Further, they could serve as model programs for the federal government.

A more extreme option is California, which has begun manufacturing insulin on its own and distributing it at very low cost. Insulin is crucial for maintaining the health of many people with diabetes, but its price has increased dramatically over the past several years. Seeing the effects on the health and finances of its citizens, the government of California has embarked on simply doing the manufacturing itself (Mullin, 2022).

The pharmaceutical industry has not, and will not, be passive and will attempt to circumvent any legislation. For example, when drugs begin to near the termination of their patents, minor reformulations can be used to extend exclusive marketing rights. Or the drug manufacturer can license the generics, or produce the less-expensive versions of the drugs themselves. All the while, "Big Pharma" continues to lobby to maintain its position in the medical care system, and to preserve its ability to charge what the market will bear for drugs.

Central controls

The major alternative to competition is imposing central controls, implying a stronger role for government. For example, the United Kingdom, with the vast majority of health spending coming through the NHS and a single budget, has been more successful than most other countries in controlling healthcare costs. It has been able to create slower increases in healthcare costs than in most other countries while still maintaining relatively good health outcomes—better than those in the United States for most standard indicators.

Table 8.11: Selected recommendations for reducing health costs, National Conference of State Legislatures

	Example
1. Administrative Simplification	All insurers use same forms and codes
2. Global Payment to Health Providers	One pre-payment for each episode of disease
3. Comprehensive Data Collection	Identify low quality and high-price providers
4. More Use of HMOs and ACOs	Integrated payments and care in these organizations
5. Performance-based Payments	Reward high value providers and procedures
6. Equalize Provider Payments	Use Medicare or Medicaid reimbursement levels
7. Reduce Drug Costs	Utilize generics; negotiate drug prices
8. Reduce Fraud	Monitor payments more closely
9. Health Promotion Disease	Target chronic diseases such as diabetes and heart
10. Emphasize Patient Safety	Reduce errors and hospital acquired infections

Source: NCSL (2011).

These central controls over spending lead directly to another of the propositions advanced by Wildavsky (2018). This argument is that there is always rationing in medical care. The question is what is the basis of the rationing, and is it equitable (see Leonhardt, 2009). In the United States medical care is rationed primarily by money—those with good insurance or private resources can get excellent care quickly, while those without the resources do not. In systems with more controlled budgets, such as the United Kingdom, the rationing principle appears to be time. Instead of potentially being denied care, patients may have to wait for a long time for appointments or for any procedures. While eventually receiving the service (at little or no cost) is certainly better than not receiving it, this can prolong suffering from the condition, as well as anxiety.

American state governments have been active in attempts to control costs in Medicaid, in part because health spending constitutes a larger share of their budgets than it does for the federal government, and they have fewer fiscal instruments to raise the money. Table 8.11 enumerates some of the instruments that state governments have been using to attempt to control costs, and shows state actions to control drug costs. Many of these instruments for cost control have depended more on direct control than those of the federal government. Some, however, also involve cost–shifting to the federal government or to individuals, rather than total savings in the amount of money spent on healthcare. Further, in some cases there have been experiments with rationing by deciding that Medicaid would not pay for some minor illnesses or complaints (Jacobs et al., 1999).

Conclusion

The increasing cost of medical care is the United States has been a problem for decades and, despite some slowing during the period of the pandemic, cost is likely to be a continuing problem. A good deal of the increasing costs will be driven by expansion of demand, with the elderly population increasing rapidly and with more people having insurance because of the Affordable Care Act. The strain of the pandemic on healthcare personnel is now leading to demands for significant increases in remuneration for these workers, especially nurses. And finally, technological change provides great benefits in care, albeit often at a very high price.

The tools that governments in the United States have for reducing expenditures are relatively weak. Some that could be the most powerful, for example negotiating drug prices for Medicare, are in fact specifically denied to government. Producing cost containment is likely to require much more direct intervention by the federal government, and the state governments, and that is not palatable to many Americans who want lower health costs but also want a less intrusive government. This may be yet another of the many trade-offs that exist within health policy, and that make developing effective and popular solutions so difficult.

The study of costs and cost containment also makes the trade-offs among the important properties of healthcare systems very evident. Many of the efforts to reduce costs may reduce access, especially when measured in time. If there are fewer MRIs then waiting times will be longer. There may also be effects of quality. If drug companies earn less money then perhaps they will invest less in new medicines that can cure dread diseases. It is difficult to argue that the amount of money now spent on medical care in the United States is not excessive, but cuts in the amount spent may impose other costs.

9

The quality of healthcare: how good is it?

The third major variable in healthcare is the quality of the care provided. In Chapter 1 I pointed out that, if we examine major indicators of the quality of care, the United States does not appear to perform well. Indicators of major health outcomes such as infant mortality, life expectancy and total mortality are all worse than most other wealthy countries. I also pointed out that some of the differences among countries is a function of social factors such as inequality and poverty, and behavioral factors (see Spencer and Grace, 2016). This chapter will attempt to focus on the quality of health services directly, as well as possible remedies for deficiencies in those services when there is a clear case that they are not performing as they should.

Defining health quality is not an easy task. Although medicine is a science, it is not always an exact science. When delivering healthcare, professionals have to deal with a highly variable input—patients—and therefore their best solutions available may not always be as effective as expected for all patients. Patients not only have variable reactions to treatments, but some may be more willing to follow the directions of their physicians than are others. Further, some patients may be more able to follow instructions, that is they can afford all of their medicines, and they understand the instructions being given. Other patients may be willing to follow directions and understand the directions, but do not have the resources to purchase all the medications they need. These interactions between the providers and the patients can be crucial in creating health outcomes, and can dilute the effects of even the best medical care.

While some standard indicators of healthcare quality, including infant mortality and life expectancy, are influenced heavily by social and economic factors,[1] others are more directly linked to the quality of care. For example, cancer survival rates can say a great deal about the quality of healthcare. Table 9.1 shows changes in the five-year survival rates for three common cancers in the United States from 1975 to 2013. Each of these three shows substantial increases in the survival rates of cancer patients, with one—pancreatic cancer—tripling. There is very high quality medicine available to patients, but perhaps not to all patients, as was shown in Chapter 7.

The above evidence is positive and, when compared with evidence from other wealthy democracies, the results are equally positive. Table 9.2 shows survival rates in wealthy and middle-income countries for all cancers, with the United States outperforming all save one of the members of this association of wealthy nations. While the overall rates of survival of cancer are very good in the United States, those outcomes are not distributed equally. Both the incidence of cancer and the death rate are higher among Black Americans, although there has been a more rapid rate of improvement among Black Americans (Giaquinto et al., 2022). Black Americans tend to live in areas with higher pollution, to have less healthy diets,

Table 9.1: Five-year cancer survival rates, United States

	1975	1985	1995	2000	2005	2010	2013
Breast	75.3	78.5	86.8	89.5	90.7	91.1	91.8
Lung	11.5	13.2	13.4	14.6	17.6	19.6	22.1
Pancreatic	3.1	3.3	3.7	5.3	6.4	9.7	11.6

Source: National Cancer Institute, SEER Program.

Table 9.2: Five-year cancer survival rates by country, 2022

	Type of Cancer		
	Breast	Stomach	Lung
United States	88.6	29.1	18.7
Brazil	87.4	24.9	18.0
France	86.9	27.7	13.6
Finland	86.6	25.2	12.3
Australia	86.2	27.9	15.0
Sweden	86.2	23.2	15.6
Canada	85.8	24.8	17.3
Germany	85.3	31.6	16.2
Japan	84.7	54.0	30.0
Denmark	82.0	17.9	11.3
United Kingdom	81.1	18.5	9.6
Poland	74.1	18.6	13.4
India	60.4	18.7	9.6

Source: CONCORD Programme, London School of Hygiene and Tropical Medicine, https://csg.lshtm.ac.uk/research/themes/concord-programme/.

and not to receive as aggressive screening as do white Americans, and for those and a number of other reasons experience higher rates of death from cancer.

The relative success in dealing with cancer, however, is not mirrored in the outcomes of the COVID-19 pandemic, with the United States having by far the highest per capita death rate of any of these wealthy nations, and indeed much higher than the death rates in numerous poorer countries (Table 9.3). By March, 2022 over one million people had died from COVID-19 in the United States. Again, these deaths were not distributed equally across the population, but occurred at a high rate among minority group members and older people. The deaths also occurred in higher numbers among people who, for whatever reason, had not been vaccinated despite the easy availability of the vaccine across the country.

These several sets of indicators intimate several things about the healthcare system of the United States. The first is that the quality of care for serious diseases such as cancer is excellent (provided, of course, the patient has good access to that care). The second is that the US health system may not be so good at dealing with public

Table 9.3: Death rates from COVID-19 (per one million population)

	US	UK	Italy	Sweden	France	Egypt	Vietnam	Peru
Deaths	2,955	2,373	2,592	1,731	2,131	230	415	6,261

Source: Worldometer Covid, https://www.worldometers.info/coronavirus/#news.

health issues, and the control of infectious diseases, as it is in dealing with acute care issues. And, finally, there is very high quality medical care available within the American healthcare system, but it is not evenly distributed. I have already shown some of the disparities of access that exist within the system, and these data demonstrate that there are also disparities in the outcomes experienced by patients.

Other measures of health quality have less to do with health outcomes and more to do with the process of delivering services to patients. One standard issue of this sort is waiting times. How long does a patient have to wait before they can see a physician, or have a CT scan, or have an elective surgery? On some measures of this sort, the United States does rather poorly. For example, in a study by the Commonwealth Foundation the United States was second worst among a group of wealthy democracies in the ability of a patient to get an answer to a question on the same day from their regular doctor's office (Table 9.4). On the other hand, in the same survey patients in the United States had among the shortest waiting times to see specialists.

These two seemingly contradictory sets of answers to a patient survey also provide some information about the American healthcare system. The first is that most doctors, and perhaps especially primary care physicians, are under a great deal of time pressure, and therefore may not provide answers quickly. On the other hand, there is perhaps a disproportionate number of specialists in the US medical system, and it is easier to get to see one given the concentration of a good deal of medical talent in specialities. Once again, the picture of quality is somewhat mixed.

Medical errors and other threats to quality

The evidence concerning outcomes for cancer patients and COVID-19 patients is important, as is the information about waiting times. We also, however, should examine more closely the day-to-day operations of the healthcare system to identify where the quality that should exist within that system may not be present. This healthcare system, or rather this collection of multiple actors interacting in complex and sometimes unpredictable manners attempting to provide healthcare, treats millions of patients each year in a wide range of settings. Given the magnitude of activities being undertaken, as well as their technical complexity, some error is inevitable. The questions are, however, how much error, what are its sources, and how can it be corrected?

How much error?

The easy answers to this question are: a great deal; and, too much. The available evidence is that errors are relatively common, occurring in diagnoses, treatments

Table 9.4: Waiting times by country

	Hear Back From a GP[1]	Get to See a Specialist[2]
Canada	33	61
United States	28	27
Sweden	24	52
Norway	22	61
United Kingdom	21	41
Australia	14	39
Netherlands	13	25
Germany	13	25
Switzerland	12	23

[1] Percent waiting more than one day.
[2] Percent waiting more than one month.
Source: Commonwealth Fund, https://www.commonwealthfund.org/publications/surveys/2021/oct/comparing-nations-timeliness-and-coordination-health-care.

and prevention. Some of these errors may be a minor inconvenience for the patient, while others can cause major medical problems or even death. The extent of the impact and deaths is debatable, with popular media and some professional sources making claims that medical errors may cause as many as 440,000 deaths per year (see Mazer and Nabhan, 2019). While the actual numbers are certainly below that, there are still thousands of iatrogenic deaths each year. The National Academy of Sciences has also reported that errors contributed to roughly 10 percent of all deaths in hospitals, as revealed in post–mortem examinations.

While deaths as a result of medical errors are obviously an extreme negative outcome of the healthcare system, there may be other less serious, but still important, negative outcomes. Patients who experience errors may spend additional time in hospital, or may require additional treatments or, worse, may lose organs or limbs. These types of medical errors are more common and one estimate by the National Academy of Sciences is that most Americans will experience some sort of medical error in their lifetimes. Another study found that 5 percent of Americans are misdiagnosed as outpatients each year (Whiteman, 2014).

The United States does not perform well when the rate of medical errors is compared with those in other comparable countries. Data collected by the Commonwealth Fund shows that over 12 percent of Americans reported problems with medication or other treatments within the past two years, (Table 9.5). This is only 1 percent greater than the average of comparable countries, but 25 percent higher than the best performing country (the Netherlands). There is no evidence about the severity of the mistakes, or their consequences, but there are a large number of mistakes being experienced by US patients.

The rates at which medical errors occur are influenced by a number of factors. As with so many aspects of healthcare, race and gender play a significant role

Table 9.5: Patients reporting medication or treatment errors within past two years, 2020 (in percent)

Australia	13.1
Sweden	12.6
United States	12.6
Germany	12.1
Switzerland	11.8
Comparable Country Average	11.4
United Kingdom	11.0
Canada	10.4
France	10.3
Netherlands	9.7

Source: Commonwealth Fund, https://www.commonwealthfund.org/series/international-health-policy-surveys.

(Singh et al., 2013; see also Box 9.1). These errors are part of a larger general category related to poor communications between providers and patients, with issues arising from some failures of both parties involved. Age also plays a factor in diagnostic errors, both for the old and the young. Diseases may present differently in elderly patients than in others and, as already noted, there are relatively few trained geriatricians in the United States. Further, providers may dismiss complaints from younger patients, assuming that they are basically healthy. Finally, errors are often attributable to misunderstanding "lifestyle" issues for patients, and assuming that symptoms are a function of drugs or alcohol, rather than of another disease.

Box 9.1: Sources of diagnostic errors

Representativeness Bias	Assuming that because a patient presents with certain familiar symptoms they must have a common condition.
Base Rate Neglect	Ignoring the prevalence of pathologies, especially based on demographic characteristics of the patient. This source of error is to some extent the opposite of the representativeness bias.
Over-confidence Bias	Physicians are skilled professionals who may assume that their diagnosis and judgment are almost always correct.
Anchoring	Once an initial diagnosis has been made, the physician may be reluctant to change it, even in the face of negative evidence.
Availability Bias	The choice of diagnosis based on information that is readily available. For example, in 2021, there may have been a tendency to assume many symptoms represented COVID-19 because it was so much in the news.
Search-Satisficing	Premature closure of the search for a diagnosis, and accepting a diagnosis too easily.

Over-diagnosis is a somewhat more subtle form of misdiagnosis (Macy, 2020). Providers may feel they are under pressure to make some diagnosis for patients who appear in their offices, and therefore may generate a diagnosis. This can also be related to defensive practice (discussed later in this chapter), with doctors wanting to minimize their probability of being sued for malpractice. This over-diagnosis may then lead to over-treatment. No medical intervention is completely safe, so the more treatments that there are, the more likely is some harm occurring for the patient.

There is also a problem of over-treatment, willfully done by doctors, whether out of ego or out of financial incentives. In fee-for-service medicine the financial rewards come from treating rather than from being more conservative in the approach to disease. There are some egregious cases of doctors, perhaps especially surgeons (Outcalt, 2021), over-treating, but it may be difficult to make a definitive case that there has been unnecessary surgery in many cases. These decisions are matters of professional judgment. There are mechanisms for monitoring the extent to which individual doctors deviate from modal patterns, but even then proving that there has been malpractice is difficult.

Prevention is perhaps the principal weakness in the quality of healthcare in the United States. It is difficult to assess exactly how much difference preventative care makes to the lives of patients, but there is certainly some impact. Early detection of serious diseases such as cancer increases the longevity of patients significantly but, even when available, patients may not use these opportunities. Fewer than 75 percent of American women have had a mammogram in the past two years, for example (KFF, 2019). The Affordable Care Act emphasized preventative medicine, but there is still a great deal of effort required to make prevention available to all citizens as a means of enhancing quality.

Although prevention and routine scanning does not appear good in the United States, in some areas the system does an excellent job in preventing complications from surgery. For example, the rates of sepsis following abdominal surgery are much lower than in other comparable countries (see Table 9.6). This relative success in preventing post-operative infections for some conditions may be an effect of the Affordable Care Act and other federal legislation introducing significant penalties for hospitals with high rates of post-operative infection. Unfortunately, success in limiting other post-operative complications, for example pulmonary embolisms, does not appear to be as good (KFF, 2021).

Table 9.6: Post-operative sepsis following abdominal surgery, 2018 (in percent)

United Kingdom	4.1
Australia	4.0
Netherlands	3.6
Sweden	1.7
United States	1.0

Source: OECD, *Health Statistics*, https://www.oecd.org/health/health-data.htm.

Patient satisfaction

The assessments of health quality discussed to this point have been more or less objective, attempting to measure health outcomes such as mortality and morbidity. The performance of healthcare systems can also be assessed more subjectively, by asking citizens how satisfied they are with their providers and the service overall. This method is used for most other services and products that citizens consume, and it is being used increasingly in healthcare. The Affordable Care Act mandates that providers assess patient satisfaction and use that information in evaluating providers and facilities (Russell et al., 2015).

Using patient evaluation for medical providers is somewhat more suspect than in other "industries". Patients know they want to get well, and to feel better, but they may not know what the possible outcomes are given their condition and the current state of medical science. Patients may expect miracles, and may express dissatisfaction with outcomes that, to professionals, may be expected. That said, patients can assess more expertly if they were treated with respect, if they had to wait an excessively long time, and whether the instructions they were given were clear.

One of the unintended outcomes of the use of patient satisfaction measures in the Affordable Care Act has been a contribution to the epidemic of opioid use in the United States (Junewicz and Youngner, 2015). Patients may tell their doctors they have chronic pain and ask for opioids. Many doctors have been reluctant to receive poor ratings from patients and, therefore, have prescribed opioids for longer than they might have wanted to ordinarily. This practice leads to addiction and the legal use of opioids then becomes transformed into what is essentially illegal use of the drugs.

Billing

Billing in a healthcare system that functions as it were entirely private even if much of the funding is public is essential for understanding its functioning Errors in billing may not cause physical harm, but they can certainly cause financial problems for the patient and for insurance companies. The complexity of hospital billing in particular also means that it is difficult for most patients to decipher how they are being charged, and then to contest that billing with the hospital.

Errors in hospital and other medical billing are not infrequent. One estimate is that 80 percent of medical billing contains an error of some sort (Gooch, 2016). In addition to "normal" errors in billing, patients may be presented with surprise bills that they expected their insurance company to pay, or with outlandish charges in emergency rooms—one patient was charged $6,000 for an ice pack and a bandage (Booth, 2019). There is no available estimate of the amount of money patients will spend each year because of billing errors, but it will obviously be in the millions of dollars.

Errors in medical billing may also be more systematic, and driven by the profit motives of health providers, resulting in higher costs for health insurance companies and higher premiums for patients. The practice of "upcoding" has been shown to be widespread in medical billing, meaning that coders who determine how to charge will apply codes for more serious conditions in order to create higher payments (Bauder et al., 2017). Whether done purposefully, which would constitute fraud, or by accident, the Government Accountability Office determined in 2013 that roughly 8 percent of billing to Medicare and Medicaid was overcharging by upcoding (King, 2014).

Fraud, waste and abuse[2]

When we move from medical errors that are largely unintentional to billing errors, we begin to consider errors that are more intentional, and more driven by individual or corporate greed. There is an ongoing pattern of doctors and hospitals increasing their incomes, sometimes greatly, by fraudulent practices, and abusing their positions within the healthcare industry. Much of this fraud is directed at federal programs such as Medicare and Medicaid. This may be in part because the auditing of these programs has not been as thorough by many private insurers, and in part because the reimbursement rates for Medicaid are lower than for private insurance, perhaps creating the sense that the provider is "owed" some extra income.[3]

The amount of money lost to fraud by the federal government health programs is substantial. In 2020, the federal government lost over $100 billion to improper claims (Table 9.7). The large majority of these losses were in Medicaid, perhaps because some providers may believe the program for the medically indigent is somewhat illegitimate. The good news, however, is that the rate of improper payments in most federal programs went down from 2019, representing some improvement in financial management within the Centers for Medicare and Medicaid Services (CMS).

The improvements in detecting and preventing improper payments were in large part due to the passage of legislation in 2019 requiring increased monitoring of payments and the identification of high-risk programs and participants. The improvements were made even after CMS suspended many enforcement activities during the pandemic in order to simplify the workloads of providers faced with unusual levels of demand. This problem is far from solved, but there have been improvements in enforcement, although whether there have been any changes in the attitudes of providers remains uncertain. The issue of improper billing became

Table 9.7: Improper payment from federal programs, 2020

	Medicare Fee for Service	Medicare Part C	Medicare Part D	Medicaid	CHIP
Amount (Billion $)	25.74	16.27	0.93	86.49	4.78
Rate (%)	6.27	6.78	1.15	21.36	27.00

Source: CMS (2020).

evident again in 2022 with high levels of improper billing in Medicare (Schulte and Hacker, 2022).

State governments are also working to prevent fraud in Medicaid at that level. Each state has a Medicaid Fraud Control Unit, responsible for detection and prosecution of fraud by providers and patients. The level of fraud reported above has led many states to place more emphasis on enforcement, especially focusing on providers with unusually high levels of claims. These activities have reduced fraud at this level, and apparently have had little or no negative impact on the legitimate treatment of conditions, for example lower back pain, that are the most open to abuse (Perez and Wing, 2019).

Government is not the only participant in healthcare that suffers from fraud by practitioners and patients. The estimated losses are not as clear as for fraud in the public sector, but it would be surprising if they were not of the same order of magnitude, meaning that it would amount to several hundred billion dollars. The same sorts of practices, such as double billing, upcoding and identity theft are involved with private insurance as are found in the public sector. Given the significant role of the federal government in all healthcare, the FBI is the principal agency for detecting healthcare fraud in the private sector, although state governments are also active.

We need to remember also that healthcare fraud is not just about the money. Unethical providers may persuade patients to undergo unnecessary procedures to earn more money, thus endangering the patients. Marketing health supplements with little or no medical value is not only expensive but may delay patients from seeking more effective treatments (see Chapter 6). And even if it were only about the money, fraud involves diverting funds that could have been put to better use, whether in healthcare or elsewhere.

Controlling and improving quality

Having detailed some of the quality issues that arise in American healthcare, the instruments available for control or punishment should also be discussed. In the best case the quality control mechanisms would not only detect errors, and perhaps punish any malfeasance, but also create some deterrence against future malfeasance, and opportunities for learning. Unfortunately, what is perhaps the major instrument for coping with quality issue is focused primarily on punishment and some restitution for the patient affected. Other mechanisms do, however, provide some ways of learning about improvements.

Licensing and accreditation

The first line of defense for health quality are the licensing and accreditation processes that assess the fitness of individuals and institutions to provide care to patients. The licensing and accreditation function is a mixed public and private activity. For example, state medical boards[4] issue licenses to physicians and nurses based on examinations and their formal degrees, but do so on behalf of medical societies that tend to control the practice of medicine, including medical education and training.

Hospitals and other medical facilities are also licensed and inspected by public as well as private organizations. Hospitals and many nursing homes are accredited by private associations such as the Joint Commission on the Accreditation of Healthcare Organizations and the Utilization Review Accreditation Commission. These accreditations are required to receive reimbursement from some health insurance programs and generally also to be licensed by state authorities. Other healthcare organizations, such as health maintenance organizations and free-standing surgical centers are accredited by other organizations.

One of the important issues in licensing in the United States is the licensing of foreign medical graduates. Medical schools in the United States do not graduate a sufficient number of physicians for the needs of the country, and therefore a significant number of practitioners who attend medical school elsewhere come to practice in the United States. These physicians play important roles in providing care in certain specialties and in underserved areas of the United States. Approximately one-quarter of all physicians in the United States now have medical degrees from foreign medical schools, The quality of the training in those foreign schools may vary, so states impose additional testing (the United States Medical Licensing Examination) and residency requirements on these graduates.

While these licensing and accrediting organizations are generally very rigorous and set high standards, we must still be aware that this is, to a great extent, self-regulation of these providers (Bauchner et al., 2015). Thus, as regulators familiar with the difficulties of providing medical care, they may be more forgiving of some deficiencies than might an outsider looking at the facilities from a completely objective position. On the other hand, however, who knows more about providing medical care than other medical providers, so the expertise of the regulators may outweigh any tendency to accept what might in some contexts appear to be substandard performance.

Evidence-based medicine and utilization

Medicine is a science, if in some ways an inexact science. It is built on basic sciences such as physiology, anatomy, microbiology and the like, and also has a huge volume of evidence based on the experience of practitioners (and their patients). There is, however, some evidence that doctors in the United States do not pay sufficient attention to the available evidence when deciding on treatments for patients. Some of this resistance to evidence can be argued to be the result of financial incentives to treat even in cases when the efficacy of the treatment is marginal. And some may be because of resistance to new procedures and treatments that are less familiar to the physicians.

The tendency to over-treat and the resistance of evidence about treatment has serious consequences for the quality of care in the United States. John E. Wennberg (2010) divided the services provided to patients into three categories: effective care, preference-sensitive care and supply-sensitive care. The first category, as the name implies, is care for which there is evidence that this is effective and better than alternative interventions. Preference-sensitive care is care for which there is no clear superior form of treatment. Finally, supply-sensitive care includes treatment for which the supply of services—hospital beds, surgeons' time, etc.—tends to determine its use.

Wennberg's analysis of the treatments being given to Medicare patients was that about 15 percent was effective care, 25 percent was preference-sensitive and 60 percent was supply-sensitive. If this breakdown of services is anywhere near correct, then the care being offered to Medicare patients at that time was very likely to include many decisions made because of the desire to utilize the capacity existing within the medical system. This analysis is corroborated by evidence that the prevalence of certain types of treatment, for example hysterectomies, is correlated with the number of providers available.

Here is another instance in which two of the three major criteria I have been applying to healthcare may come into conflict. They will conflict when the choice of newer procedures and medications that are indeed superior than older ones are selected and impose higher costs. These two criteria also align. Cost and quality as criteria for assessing healthcare systems do align when we think of over-treatment, and over-testing. Not only can that testing and treatment harm the patient, but it also imposes unnecessary costs on the patient (and the healthcare system as a whole). Likewise, a physician who chooses to continue to prescribe an older medication that is still effective is reducing cost when compared to one who prescribes a newer medication that may also be effective but is more expensive.[5]

Patashnik et al. (2017) use the evidence from Wennberg's study and a number of other studies to question the extent to which the American healthcare system is, as in one model discussed in Chapter 1, the best in the world. They demonstrate that doctors and medical societies are slow to adopt innovations, even when there is ample evidence to support those innovations. The cause for this slow adoption of innovation may be venal, and related to a desire to maximize income, it may be inertia, or it may be because the time pressures on contemporary physicians make learning new techniques more difficult. For whatever reason, this does mean that the delivery of healthcare services is not as advanced technically as it should be.[6]

Sanctioning providers

For individual providers in healthcare the principal quality control mechanism is the professional association, such as the medical society or its equivalent in each state. These organizations are responsible for the initial licensing of physicians as well as determining whether those licenses should be revoked. Physicians may be sanctioned for a variety of reasons, with the most common being inappropriate writing of prescriptions, especially for opioids. This was a major reason for actions against doctors before the opioid crisis, but has become more common. Another common reason for removing licenses is alcohol or drug abuse by the physician.

There is relatively little sanctioning of physicians because of incompetency. Not only are other physicians reluctant to declare their colleagues incompetent to practice, but the standards of proof of incompetence are rather high, meaning that licensing boards may not want to invest the time and resources into marginal cases. This reluctance means that, rather than being removed from practice proactively, it may be up to the malpractice system (see below) to detect and punish most incompetent physicians. It is difficult to obtain comprehensive information on the number who lose licenses, but one example would be Pennsylvania in 2021 where six physicians lost their license to practice (Pennsylvania Department of State, 2022).

Another means of improving quality is to provide monetary incentives to maintain or improve quality. These monetary incentives are primarily in the form of punishment for poor performance. For example, Medicare imposes a 1 percent penalty on hospitals that have high rates of infections and avoidable complications, as well as for hospital readmissions (Rau, 2021). In extreme cases Medicare and Medicaid may terminate their contract with hospitals that continue to have high levels of adverse events (see, for example, Mucio, 2022). In other cases, hospitals may be, in essence, fined by insurers for high levels of additional costs resulting from errors or poor treatment.

Cultural change

Rather than focusing on culpability and punishment as incentives to improve quality, cultural change within providing organizations can be used to emphasize quality and change behaviors (de Bienassis et al., 2020). These types of changes within healthcare have been fostered by both private and public organizations. Among the private sector actors, the Joint Commission on the Accreditation of Healthcare Organizations has been a major player. Beginning at least a decade before this writing, the Joint Commission has emphasized patient safety as a major component of their accreditation process (Chassin and Loeb, 2013).

In doing this, the Joint Commission emphasized a culture of safety, and also attempted to move healthcare organizations away from a culture of blame and punishment. In part the emphasis on blame tended to move the safety question to ex post monitoring—trying to detect errors and unsafe practices after they had occurred. This approach obviously is inferior to a strategy of preventing errors in the first place. Making that change in culture in hospitals and other organizations has also involved changing thinking about the sources of error. The traditional model has been to focus on the individual, while many problems in safety for patients are more systemic (Govindarajan et al., 2019).

Malpractice as a remedy

Malpractice suits are the most commonly used means of addressing medical errors in the United States. These are in essence tort proceedings conducted in civil court, arguing that the medical practitioner in question injured the patient in some

Table 9.8: Elements of a malpractice case

A Duty of Care is Owed
That Duty was Breached
The Breach Caused Harm
Some Identifiable Linkage
Deviation from Accepted Standards
Real Damage
Burden of Proof on the Plaintiff
Statute of Limitations

way. The elements of malpractice are presented in Table 9.8. The harm done to the patient does not have to be intentional, and indeed almost never is, but there may still be damage because of negligence or a lack of skill, or just poor luck. As shown in the table, the assumption is that there is a duty of care on behalf of the provider and that duty is breached.

Malpractice is big business and involves big money. Although there is variance by year, there is an average of 85,000 malpractice cases in the United States each year. From 2010 to 2019 an average of $4.2 billion was paid out to patients who won their cases, for an average of almost $250,000. The costs for doctors are also substantial, although also highly variable. For example, surgeons in New York often pay over $100,000 per year in insurance premiums, while family practitioners may pay only $5,000 in some states. In general, surgeons, anesthesiologists and obstetricians pay the highest rates for malpractice insurance.

Malpractice suits are not rare events in the lives of physicians. It is estimated that 75 percent of physicians in low-risk specialties, for example dermatology or family practice, will face a malpractice suit at some time during their careers, and that almost 100 percent of those in high-risk specialties such as surgery will be sued. Women physicians are significantly less likely to be sued than are male physicians, regardless of the speciality, but are still sued frequently. Because malpractice suits are widespread, they exert a pervasive influence over the behavior of physicians and other medical practitioners.

The premiums that physicians pay for malpractice insurance become a component of the prices they charge their patients. But those premiums are not the only contribution that concerns about malpractice make to the bills received by patients. The most important additional cost is from defensive practice (Bovbjerg et al., 1996), meaning that the physicians order additional tests for patients just to make sure that nothing is missed in a diagnosis. The doctor may be confident that there is nothing seriously wrong with the patient, but still orders the additional tests for fear that, if something is missed and the patient is seriously ill, they will be sued for malpractice. Although estimates vary, it seems that defensive practice adds at least $40–45 billion to healthcare costs each year (Sullivan, 2018).

If a plaintiff wins a malpractice case, the award may have two components. The first is real economic damages. If the successful plaintiff cannot work any longer, or cannot work as effectively as before the medical error, how much income will he or she lose as a result of the error, or also how much did they lose while recovering from the mistreatment? The second component is for pain and suffering, otherwise conceptualized as punitive damages. These awards may be awarded by a jury or by a judge, with the pain and suffering component often having been much larger than the actual damages, and also being the cost that drives attempts to control malpractice awards.

Malpractice is usually associated with physicians, but other providers in healthcare can also be subject to these suits. Indeed, in the case of a recent death caused by an error in dosage of a medication, a nurse was convicted of negligent homicide (Medina, 2022). Further, pharmaceutical companies and the makers of healthcare products, for example baby powder, face class-action suits from individuals who have been harmed by those products. The healthcare industry is thus characterized by a great deal of legal and financial peril for those involved in providing products and services.

While the malpractice may appear to be a poor way to hold the medical establishment accountable for their actions, it does have at least one major virtue. It, and the product liability suits mentioned above, provides patients who may not have many financial resources the opportunity to gain compensation for damages. Malpractice cases are handled by lawyers on a contingency basis—if they lose the lawyers receive no fee, but if they win they may receive up to 40 percent of the award. This also provides something of a constraint on the lawyers—they have to think carefully before taking a marginal case if they will have to invest time and other resources.[7]

Malpractice reform

The costs of malpractice insurance, and their effects on total medical costs, have led to a number of attempts to reform this component of the legal system. The ideas for reforms range from rather simple modifications of the existing system to more complete overhauls of the malpractice system. Few of the more radical reforms have been attempted, given the extent to which lawyers (most legislators are lawyers) defend the system, and its capacity to provide redress to citizens who have experienced harm while receiving medical care. There have, however, been a number of efforts to implement less sweeping reforms.

The most common reform of malpractice has been to limit the awards that can be given to patients. As of the end of 2021, over half of the states had set a limit on the awards possible in a malpractice case. Ten other states have attempted to cap awards, but those laws have been deemed to violate states' constitutions and could not be enforced. Also, during the Trump administration the federal government tried unsuccessfully to limit the awards in malpractice cases. The limitations were thrown out because they violated equal protection principles—why limit one type of tort award?—or because they violated the power of juries to make their own decisions on awards (Padget, 2003).

In most instances the limits to awards are for non-economic rewards, for pain and suffering, disfigurement, etc. Economic awards for real losses from the mistreatment by the medical system are not limited, and the same is generally true for punitive damages. The US Supreme Court has ruled,[8] however, that generally punitive damages cannot be greater than nine times actual economic damages. These caps help to solve some of the economic issues of malpractice for doctors, but may not address some of the problems that plaintiffs may encounter with slow proceedings and long delays in receiving needed funds.

The initial findings after the reduction of awards in some states has been that malpractice insurance rates have gone down, and total medical spending in the states has also gone down (Paik et al., 2013; Born et al., 2017). In addition, there were fewer malpractice cases brought to court, and the number of physicians entering "risky" specialties such as obstetrics was increased. What did not appear to change, however, was the amount of defensive practice, with physicians continuing to order large numbers of tests that may not have been indicated by the symptoms of patients.

Another possible reform of malpractice would be to move the standard for awarding damages from contributory negligence to comparative fault. In the former system for assigning blame, it is essentially all or nothing. One side or the other is more at fault, and if the physician is deemed more at fault they are obliged to pay for all the damages. For example, even if a patient contributed to a poor outcome from a surgery by not following the instructions given by the surgeon, if a mistake produced most of the harm then the surgeon is liable for all the damages. With comparative fault, the patient could have recovered only some of the costs, hence reducing the amount of the settlement and total malpractice costs.

More radical reforms of malpractice could include the changes listed in Table 9.9. The majority of these reforms attempt to move away from an adversarial proceeding in court to administrative or mediated solutions. This movement away from an adversarial relationship may be less expensive for the healthcare providers and reduce total medical costs. The outcomes of an administrative proceeding can also be more certain for the patient. For example, implementing the *res ipsa* doctrine would mean that if something went wrong in a treatment, then the facts speak for themselves, and the patient is entitled to some compensation.

Malpractice is not likely to disappear as the principal means of holding doctors and other health providers accountable for their actions. It is crucial to maintain accountability for providers and it appears especially important to retain the access to redress that having contingency fees for malpractice provides. That said, the process can be improved and some of the more egregious elements within the system can be eliminated. Further, this system of accountability does perpetuate the culture of blame that other actors concerned with quality in healthcare are attempting to eliminate.

Table 9.9: Possible reforms of malpractice system

1. "No fault" payments for harms, with set payments

2. *Res ipsa loquitur* assessment of harm, with set payments

3. "Safe harbor"—no malpractice claim possible if procedures adhered to

4. Administrative determinations of awards for damages

5. Mediation, with recourse to court system

6. Arbitration

Conclusion

Consistent with one of the images of American healthcare discussed in Chapter 1, some aspects of American healthcare are indeed of very high quality. Treatments for major diseases such as cancer appear to be very effective, and infection prevention is also good. What US healthcare often most notably falls down on are the routine matters of primary care and preventative medicine. The culture of healthcare has been oriented toward the hospital and high-tech care, rather than the more mundane, yet crucial, aspects of care provided by primary care physicians.

Although it is valuable as a means of allowing individuals who may have been harmed within the healthcare system to seek redress, even if they do not have the resources to hire a lawyer, malpractice as a major means of dealing with quality presents problems. This method of accountability imposes more costs on the healthcare system through insurance premiums and defensive practice, and focuses on punishment rather than prevention. There are other mechanisms of control in place, but much of the emphasis on improving quality remains vested in malpractice.

American healthcare is good—remember that the comparisons used throughout the book are to other wealthy countries with excellent healthcare. One of the reasons for the relatively poor performance may be that not everyone in the United States has access to the care that is available, and therefore the averages are not as good. However, given the huge amounts of money being spent on healthcare, some solution to that problem should be possible. This will be discussed in the next chapter.

10

What's next? Continuing health reform after the Affordable Care Act

The Affordable Care Act (ACA) was a milestone, but for many health policy experts, and for many citizens, it is only one milestone on a long journey toward an even more comprehensive version of health insurance for all Americans. Even after the implementation of the ACA, including the expansion of Medicaid, there are approximately 30 million Americans who lack any health insurance (as of 2022), and there are millions of additional people who are underinsured. And many citizens who do have health insurance are disappointed in how high the premiums and out-of-pocket payments are, and struggle to make good use of their insurance because of co-payments and deductibles.

While getting as much of the population as possible fully insured for healthcare is the major goal for any continuing reforms of the healthcare system, this is not the only issue that should concern those responsible for American health policy. There are other major issues, such as the continuing high cost of care and the deficiencies in the system that were exposed by the COVID-19 outbreak, that also require attention. The ACA has been a battle won, but there is still a war going on.

Expanding access

The question then is what is next on the agenda for health policy, and more specifically how will access be improved? Taking the continuation of coverage under the ACA as a given, there are at least four options for reform, ranging from incremental adjustments in the ACA to an almost complete overhaul of the health insurance system. These options were debated in part in the 2020 presidential campaign, especially in the Democratic primaries. Progressives, notably Senator Bernie Sanders (I-VT), were advocating the more extreme reforms, while others, such as (now) President Biden, were advocating more moderate change. But, although there is no interest in repealing the ACA, there was little support in the Democratic Party for simply maintaining the ACA as it is. While Republicans now appear resigned to the survival of Obamacare, they are certainly not supportive of any movements toward more publicly provided health insurance coverage, and keep discussing private alternatives such as health savings accounts.

First, there are options for reforming the ACA to make it more inclusive and also more cost-effective. One option to address cost issues would be to cap the reimbursements made by private insurers through ACA policies at the rates paid by Medicare or Medicaid, or somewhere between the two (Blumberg et al., 2020). The same caps might be applied to all private insurance, but that regulatory authority might be more clearly in the hands of the states than the federal government.

The principal reform that could affect both access and cost would be to restore the individual mandate that was repealed by the Trump administration in 2017. If the risk pool for ACA policies were expanded to include more younger, healthier people then this should keep price increases of the policies in check, while also ensuring that more people were covered. Although perhaps not as effective, some of the same goals could be achieved by using carrots—incentives for buying an insurance policy—rather than sticks—penalties for not being covered—when dealing with the uninsured population.

Another approach to reform within the context of the existing system would be to allow individuals to buy into Medicaid or perhaps Medicare. This would assume that the buy-in price would be lower than that of private insurance purchased through the exchanges, or that the coverage would be better than those individual policies, or both. Deciding on the correct pricing structure would be difficult, but this plan could benefit individuals, and it might also benefit the public insurance programs because they would have a broader risk pool. This would be especially beneficial for Medicare, but could also benefit Medicaid, of which a large number of people with chronic and disabling conditions are clients.

Some economists have argued that the issues of access and cost can be addressed through some seemingly simple regulations. The current healthcare insurance system tends to produce prices for group insurance that are lower than individual prices if an individual purchases a policy. If all insured, regardless of how they acquired insurance, were to have the same (lower) rate it would make it easier to expand coverage (Colander, 2017). This would mean in essence creating one big risk pool regardless of how insurance is purchased.

The incremental option for moving beyond the ACA is to create a public option within the existing set of insurance options offered through the exchanges. The federal government would create a plan (or more likely four plans corresponding to the Bronze, Silver, Gold and Platinum options of ACA policies) that would be available to anyone who visited the exchanges looking for health insurance. The likelihood is that the public plan would be cheaper than the private plans for the same coverage, simply because the federal government would not have high-priced executives running the program, nor would it be paying for extensive advertising for the plan.[1]

A mid-range option for reform would be "Medicare for All". The basic idea would be that anyone who wanted to could enroll in Medicare, without having to wait to reach 65 years of age. This plan might be the simplest administratively, given that the program already exists, but it may not be as simple as it appears. In the first place, Medicare insurance does not meet all the criteria that plans offered through the ACA must meet, so there might be a need for "Medigap" insurance for anyone who signed up. And Medicare is not inexpensive. Some of that high cost might be reduced if the risk pool were expanded to include younger, healthier people, but the adjustment might take some time.

Finally, there are discussions of a "single-payer" plan that would make the federal government the sole insurer, or close to the sole insurer, for the entire population. This plan would be analogous to the national insurance plans that exist in other wealthy democracies. Implementing this plan would be difficult, and would involve doing things such as essentially putting major health insurance companies (which are also major lobbyists) out of business, with the loss of millions of jobs. Many of those who would lose their jobs might be hired by government to deal with the expanded workload of the Department of Health and Human Services, but there would still be huge transaction costs. The question would be whether those costs could be offset by the benefits of a national plan.

Politically, it is interesting to see the extent to which some form of national health insurance program has become a part of normal discourse, at least among Democrats and Independents (Draper, 2019). Much of this movement toward a more progressive approach to healthcare has come about because of the relentless pressures from individuals such as Senator Sanders and RoseAnn DeMoro, former head of the National Nurses Union. But the Democratic Party has also learned that there is a strong desire on the part of the American public for something that can improve access and lower costs to individuals within the healthcare system. As Bernie Sanders' pollster said, "If people are talking about health care, we are winning" (Draper, 2019, 34).

Public option

The first of the possible extensions of the role of the federal government in healthcare would be to create a public option within the ACA exchanges (Neuman et al., 2919). To provide this option the federal government would have to begin to operate as an insurance company of sorts. That would be far from unprecedented, since there are already a number of federal insurance programs in existence,[2] but this insurance operation would require perhaps more thorough planning and risk assessment.

The public option was proposed during the run-up to the 2008 presidential election by President Obama, then a candidate. The option appeared in several early proposals for legislation to provide healthcare coverage, but was left out of the final legislation because of the threat of a filibuster that would have killed the legislation (CNN, 2009). Since that time, the public option has reappeared in political debates several times. Hillary Clinton proposed it in the 2016 presidential campaign, and Joe Biden advocated it in the 2020 campaign. By 2020 this became seen as the most conservative option for continued healthcare reform (at least by Democrats) when it was compared to Medicare for All, or a single-payer plan.

While the public option was sold politically as a less extreme option than Medicare for All, it could still be used to move the healthcare system toward a single-payer plan of some sort. It has been argued that one scenario for the public option would be to attempt to dominate the insurance market. Because of the lower overhead expenses that the public organization, or perhaps a contractor, would have it could afford to pay hospitals and physicians more than private insurers. To save total costs it would be unlikely to do that (see below), but it could charge its beneficiaries less than would other plans in the ACA. Those differences from the private insurers should move patients to this program, and could make it the preferred insurer for providers. Over time, it is argued, the public option could dominate the market.

Other scenarios for the public option would be to focus on cost containment rather than on dominating the market and driving out private insurers. The strategy for this version would be, as discussed for one option for reforming the ACA, to cap provider reimbursements, perhaps to the levels of Medicare reimbursements. If the policies offered by the public sector were made attractive to potential purchasers, then the increasing amount of reimbursements made with lower rates would drive down total costs of healthcare. This version of the plan would, of course, be opposed by hospitals and perhaps by physicians (Mankiw, 2009). However, as increasing numbers of physicians are becoming employees of hospitals and other institutions and receive salaries rather than fees, some of that opposition might be mitigated.

Although not a public option per se, state governments are considering creating their own health insurance programs, including options for single-payer plans within individual states (Sparer, 2019). More progressive states such as New York, Vermont or California could create their own programs for their citizens, and these might serve as models for an eventual federal single-payer plan. Vermont actually adopted a plan like this in 2011, but abandoned it three years later after the tax costs for small businesses proved to be excessive (Brinker, 2014; McDonough, 2015). However, a larger state with a more diverse economy may be able to make such a plan function, as the state of Washington may (Capretta, 2020), although the initial trials there and in Colorado have been disappointing (Reed, 2023b). Further, beginning with the states would match the incremental manner in which many reforms in US social policy have been adopted.

In summary, the development of a public option within the existing multi-payer health insurance system would give the federal government considerable leverage over access and cost. It would, however, require the federal government to develop a new insurance agency, or significantly expand the operations of existing organizations. There would also be some effects on private insurers who would lose customers, although not as great an impact as for the other options for reform. As with all the options for reform, this option will depend on the relative strengths of the political parties in Washington.

Medicare for all

The phrase "Medicare for All" has become something of a shorthand for a single-payer plan, as well as a political slogan.[3] Some advocates do really talk about taking the existing Medicare program and allowing anyone to buy into the program the same way they might buy a private insurance policy. This goes back at least to a proposal made by Elijah Cummings in the early twenty-first century, and remains a possibility. Several bills have been proposed in Congress that would have expanded Medicare, for example H. R. 1384 (2019), and that specific option will be discussed briefly, along with an option for buying into Medicaid, before the chapter goes on to discuss a more generic version of the single-payer plan.

In some ways, extending Medicare to the entire population might not be such a good deal for people, except for those who could get health insurance in no other way. As already discussed in Chapter 3, Medicare costs its beneficiaries a good deal of money each year in premiums and co-insurance payments. Most legislation proposed in Congress would eliminate the co-pays and deductibles, but were rather vague about the funding of the program. For younger and healthier populations, some of these charges may be higher than what might be attainable on the ACA exchanges. Still, this is an existing and generally efficient health insurance program that could be extended with minimal difficulties. Further, if the risk pool is extended it could drive downward coinsurance costs for all insured persons.

One of the political problems that the idea of extending Medicare for all raises is what would that do for the coverage of those seniors who already receive their medical insurance through the program? The fear voiced by some current recipients is that expanding the program would undermine their coverage and weaken the special place that Medicare has had in the healthcare system. The American Association of Retired Persons (AARP), the major lobbying group for people over 55 in the United States, supports universal health access, but in the list of programs it supports does not mention expanding Medicare, although it does support maintaining Medicaid as an entitlement program.

Another option that is discussed less frequently, but would use existing program infrastructure, would be allowing anyone to buy into Medicaid. In some ways this would be a better deal for the insured, because as it now functions there are limited co-pays and deductibles, and in most states the program has benefits that are not available in Medicare. The difficulty is that this option really would not be a single-payer plan, but rather over 50 programs when those in the territories are counted. The states would almost certainly have the option of refusing to allow purchases, and, finally, calculating an appropriate premium for joining Medicaid would be difficult. Still, this is one relatively simple way to make coverage more available.

These incremental options for reform appear relatively easy administratively, and they have a great deal of public support, even among Republicans (Table 10.1). Republicans may consider the extension of these programs the lesser of several

Table 10.1: Public support for extending Medicare and Medicaid (percent supporting)

	Total	Democrats	Independents	Republicans
Allowing individuals to buy into Medicare	77	85	75	69
Allowing individuals to buy into Medicaid	75	85	75	64

Source: Kaiser Family Foundation, *Public Opinion on Single-Payer, National Health Plans*, October 16, 2020.

possible evils (in their minds) that could emerge from attempts to reform the healthcare system. The support for buying into either Medicare or Medicaid is approximately the same, although there is less support from Republicans for buying into Medicaid, perhaps because of its identification by some as a "welfare" program.

Single-payer plan

Implementing the ACA has involved a number of actors, as is true for implementing many public programs (Pressman and Wildavsky, 1974). The various proposals for reform of the existing healthcare programs and the creation of a single-payer program that would provide essentially free care to all citizens would involve an even larger number of changes. The plans for a single-payer program would eliminate private insurance—whether overnight or phased out over several years.

Moving to a single-payer plan, whether it is gradually through a public option or more quickly through the adoption of a single-payer plan, will involve some significant transaction costs. Millions of Americans now receive their insurance through private insurers (including those getting their insurance through the ACA), so a single-payer plan run through the public sector would mean thousands of people losing their jobs. In addition, thousands of stockholders in those private firms will no longer have dividends from their stock. Those stockholders, which include a number of pension programs, would have to be compensated in some way. A single-payer plan once implemented will be more efficient and less expensive, but getting there will not be easy.

Politically, it matters very much how the single-payer plan is described (see Table 10.2). The manner in which both policy problems and policy solutions are constructed is important for their political success in getting onto an agenda and then being adopted (Barbehön, 2022). For the single-payer plan, the most acceptable label is "universal healthcare", followed closely by "Medicare for All". Predictably, the label of socialized medicine is not widely accepted among the American public. Also, the term "single-payer plan" does not appear to be well understood by the respondents to this survey, meaning that this term is best reserved for academic rather than political discourse.

Table 10.2: Terms used affect support for a national health plan (in percent)

Term	Support	Oppose	No Opinion
Universal Health Coverage	63	31	6
Medicare-for-All	63	34	3
National Health Plan	59	36	5
Single-Payer Health Insurance	49	32	19
Socialized Medicine	46	44	10

Source: Kaiser Family Foundation, *Public Opinion on Single-Payer, National Health Plans*, October 16, 2020.

Public opinion about reform

The ACA has been in effect for almost ten years, but there are still continuing pressures for change. These come to a great extent from political leaders and from experts in health policy, but the general public is also concerned about change. Some would like to prevent more public involvement in healthcare, but there is a significant majority that would like to extend public involvement and create some form of public insurance that would be available to all, or at least most, citizens. But that majority does have internal differences to making the move from the ACA to a more public version of insurance.

In 2019 three-quarters of Americans surveyed supported the federal government taking a greater role in helping citizens to obtain health insurance. That is a large majority, but it was actually down from the support in 2006 and 2008 (Table 10.4). There were minor drops in support among Democrats and Independents, but a very sharp drop in support among Republicans. That large drop appears to reflect the sentiment that the ACA was a sufficient intervention and no more was required. That desire to halt further expansion of the role of the federal government may be true to a lesser extent among the other two groups of respondents.

When asked specifically about a single-payer plan of some sort, the expansion toward something like a single-payer plan received majority support from respondents in 2017, and the levels of support have remained stable (Table 10.3). Since that time support has been averaging around 55 percent of respondents, while opposition has averaged around 43 percent. That is not, however, a very large majority of voter support to attempt to make a major change in health policy. This is especially true given the differences in support between the parties, with 94 percent of Democrats favoring the proposal in 2019, while 60 percent of Republicans still opposed it (Table 10.4).

Although support for greater government involvement in healthcare is not particularly strong, there is also limited confidence in the existing state of US healthcare. For example, in 2022 only 38 percent of the public questioned said they had a great deal or quite a lot of confidence in the medical system. This rather lukewarm support for the medical system had been more or less the same since the 1990s, but was much lower than it had been earlier. In 1975, 80 percent of the respondents to the Gallup survey reported they had great or quite a lot of confidence in the medical system.[4] This appears to have been a period in which Americans very much believed they had the best healthcare system in the world.

Table 10.3: Should the federal government be responsible for making sure that all Americans have health insurance? (in percent)

	2000	2005	2007	2009	2011	2013	2015	2017	2018	2019	2020	2021	2022
Yes	59	64	69	54	47	54	45	52	56	57	54	56	56
No	38	34	28	41	50	44	52	45	42	42	45	42	43

Source: Gallup, *Healthcare Polls*, various years.

Table 10.4: Partisan support for government doing more to provide health insurance (percent in favor)

	2006	2008	2019
Democrats	96	92	94
Independents	86	73	77
Republicans	72	49	40
Total	85	75	74

Source: Kaiser Family Foundation, *Public Opinion on Single-Payer, National Health Plans*, October 16, 2020.

Table 10.5a: Perceived benefits of single-payer plans by supporters (in percent)

	Very Important	Somewhat Important
Covers All Americans	89	9
Simplifies the Healthcare System	79	18
Eliminates Premiums	56	33
Eliminates Co-Pays and Deductibles	56	32
Shifts Payments to Taxes	45	38
Eliminates Private Health Insurance Companies	38	29

Table 10.5b: Respondents who believe they can keep existing insurance

	Yes	No	Don't Know
Supporters of Single-Payer Plan	67	24	9
Opponents of Single-Payer Plan	41	51	8

Source: Kaiser Family Foundation, *Public Opinion on Single-Payer, National Health Plans*, October 16, 2020.

Those who support a single-payer plan of some sort perceive a number of virtues coming from such a program (Table 10.5a). Clearly, the most important of those virtues is that such a plan will provide universal access to healthcare for citizens. This is followed closely by their desire to simplify the "jungle" that exists within healthcare. There is some bias against private insurers among the respondents, but that would not be found among those who do not favor the single-payer plan. That said, it is interesting that those who do support the plan believe that they can keep their existing coverage (Table 10.5b), while those who did not support the plan were skeptical of their ability to remain insured as they were.

Finally, we should consider the extent to which Americans consider healthcare a right, or more as something one earns by virtue of economic success, or perhaps membership in certain social groups, for example living long enough to become a senior citizen (Maruthappu et al., 2013). In 2022 well over half of Americans believed it is the responsibility of the federal government to provide healthcare, with the implication this is a right of citizenship rather than a matter of personal choice or economic circumstances.

Tireless tinkering

Most of this chapter has been about major reforms in health access, building on the successes of the ACA, and attempting to overcome some of the weaknesses of that legislation. That will be the big news in health policy if and when it occurs, but there are also a number of smaller reform issues that can and should be addressed. Although perhaps not as dramatic as moving to a single-payer plan, reforming pricing of prescription drugs, or improving equity in healthcare, can make major improvements in the system of delivering medical care, and can address the policy priorities of many citizens.

The direction of change in healthcare will depend in part on which party controls the White House and Congress. Almost all of the pressure for comprehensive reform comes from the Democratic Party and groups allied to that party. With Republican control of government, the policy options being pursued will more likely be more market based, including perhaps returning to their failed quest to repeal Obamacare. Some of the same reform dynamics may occur at the state level, with more conservative states using market-based systems or reducing commitments to healthcare more generally, while more progressive states will continue to press for a larger public dimension for healthcare.

There are also some major issues in healthcare that have not been addressed by major reform proposals. One of the more obvious of these is mental health. Although mental health disorders are widespread, there has been much less attention given to these issues than to somatic health issues. The *Dobbs* decision in 2022 made more evident the need for greater attention to reproductive healthcare. And, of course, the continuation of the COVID-19 pandemic for almost four years (at the time of publication) places continuing stress on the healthcare system.

Institutions and confidence

While access and cost are perhaps the major issues in American health policy for the near future, there are also several important institutional questions to consider. These questions have arisen to a great extent as a function of the pandemic and the strains that this major event in healthcare placed on the system. For example, the Centers for Disease Control and Prevention (CDC), which has long been a highly respected organization providing expert advice to the medical professions and to the public about communicable diseases, has come under a great deal of criticism of its handling of the COVID-19 pandemic. Some of those complaints were about the seeming indecision in the organization in offering advice, and some resulted from attempts to politicize the organization during the Trump administration (Besser, 2020).

The leadership of the CDC has recognized the need to reform its practices, given the perceived failures to respond adequately to the pandemic (LaFraniere and Weiland, 2022). It sponsored a study of the organization's performance during the crisis, and requested recommendations on how to improve performance. A number of leading experts in the field have now become involved in attempts to make the CDC a more nimble and public-friendly organization as opposed to the rather closed, scientific organization it has been.

The Food and Drug Administration (FDA) has also been a respected organization, which has been effective in regulating pharmaceuticals. Its success in preventing thalidomide from producing the same tragedies in the United States that it caused in Europe, among other things, had solidified the reputation of the organization (Carpenter, 2010). However, the controversies over vaccination, the rejection of alternative treatments, and the involvement of the organization in political conflicts have undermined the FDA and produced a need for redeveloping the reputation for probity and accuracy for the FDA.

The troubles encountered by the CDC and FDA, and the capacity to cope with possible pandemics and other medical emergencies, is perhaps the tip of the iceberg of a more general questioning of science and the medical professions. While access to health information from reliable sources such as the Mayo Clinic or Johns Hopkins University is valuable for individuals seeking to understand and manage their health problems, the amount of disinformation on the internet is presenting problems. For example, the lesser but still significant spread of the monkeypox virus is being met with the same skepticism about medical science as did the COVID-19 virus (Lewis, 2022).

Controlling costs

If the access problems for healthcare are solved through some form of single-payer plan, the problem of cost will remain. The Inflation Reduction Act of 2022 made one important step in the direction of reducing pharmaceutical costs to patients in Medicare, but this was only a beginning of what needs to be done in controlling drug costs, and costs more generally. The rise of medical costs slowed somewhat during the pandemic, but by 2022 were beginning to increase quickly again, along with rapid inflation in the economy in general.

It is important to remember that adopting a single-payer plan would be important for reducing costs as well as increasing access. A significant portion of the total costs of healthcare in the United States comes from the competition (or pseudo-competition) among the providers of health insurance and other components of the system. If those administrative overheads could be reduced with a single-payer, then estimates are that 10 percent or more of total expenditures could be eliminated (Chapter 8).

This being said, the short-term transaction costs of moving from a dominance of private insurers to a public insurer would be significant. Millions of people would have to secure insurance through the new system, and the pre-existing insurers would have to be compensated for their loss of business. Doctors and hospitals would also have to adjust their billing systems, although ultimately those would be much simpler and should involve fewer staff members. The staff lost from private insurers, or some equivalents, would have to be hired by government to manage the increased volume of claims on public insurance. In short, transition will not be painless or costless.

Leaving aside the possibilities of moving to a single-payer plan, there are still a number of less dramatic steps that could be taken to stabilize costs (Chapter 8). Many of these involve simplifying and coordinating the administrative complexities in the system; in other words overcoming the jungle. Other changes would involve going beyond the limited changes in the Inflation Reduction Act and doing something on a much larger scale with drug prices. These prices are perhaps the most vexing aspect of medical costs for patients—especially those with chronic conditions. The states have made some progress in coping with these prices, but significant progress may depend on the involvement of the federal government.

Finally, the American healthcare system needs greater attention to evidence-based policymaking. There is an immense amount of information available on how to make medical care more effective, more efficient and safer. This information is not always used as well as it might be, because of inertia, time constraints or beliefs that existing treatment modalities are as good. There is evidence that American doctors often lag behind their counterparts in other parts of the world in the adoption of innovations (Patashnik et al., 2017), and this slowness to adapt may impose higher costs and create lower quality care.

Quality

The importance of quality when thinking about the continuing reforms of the healthcare system should not be forgotten. Accessible, low-cost medical care may not be of much use if the quality of the care being delivered is not good. In some ways the issues with quality may require much less intervention by the federal government than the other two main variables discussed here. The medical professions themselves are committed to quality, although their definitions of that attribute may at times differ from that held by other actors. Further, despite its flaws, the threat of malpractice suits also places pressure on actors to maintain quality.

Although there are those strong private influences for quality, government still has a role to play in improving how the system performs. Most of the interventions are through regulations, and the outcomes of the pandemic have led to demands for closer regulation, and better communication with citizens about major health issues. Much of the negative discussion of the CDC, for example, related to the poor communication with citizens and attempts to communicate in scientific terms that were not understood by the average person.[5] Although the CDC has long had strong international connections, it appears not to have been able to keep up with the speed with which diseases, and information about them, now move (Healy, 2022).

As well as communicating with the public, governments at all levels need to prepare better for the crises that almost inevitably will arise. Governments are not the only organizations that seem to forget very easily that crises occur again and again, but their forgetfulness and failure to plan ahead are more glaring than for individuals or other organizations. The COVID-19 pandemic has been more serious than previous outbreaks, such as the swine flu and SARS, but it has been a difference of degree rather than type. In fairness, the federal government had planned for a pandemic during the Obama administration, but these plans were simply discarded by Trump (Tracy, 2020).

In the United States state and local governments also are important for planning for healthcare and other emergencies, and in general appear to be more successful than the federal government. This is true for states such as those in the South that are frequently hit by hurricanes, and those in the West that are more likely to have earthquakes and wildfires. While the states can be capable of managing problems within their own territory, that capacity may be no substitute for a more coordinated capacity to address health issues that transcend state boundaries, which almost any problem will.

Conclusion

Governments are in the business of reforming themselves and their policies. Even well-performing governments, especially democratic ones, continually attempt to make themselves perform better, and to produce better outcomes for their citizens. Health policy in the United States, despite the beliefs of some more chauvinistic citizens and egotistical providers, does not comfortably fit into the category of "well-performing" policy areas. Despite numerous reforms already implemented, some actually quite successful health policy in the United States has a very long way to go to match the achievements of the sector in other advanced democracies.

This final chapter has discussed the possible directions for future reforms. Although there is general public support for change, and even major change, advocates within the political system may find producing that change difficult. The constitutional separation of powers and the sharp partisan differences between the parties have made reform difficult. That said, the Inflation Reduction Act in 2022 did produce reforms such as (limited) negotiation of drug prices for Medicare, a reform that has been pursued for years.

Even if the large-scale shift to a single-payer plan is not possible through Congress, there are ways of producing change through executive action, or through the states, or even through the court system. Public support for a more comprehensive public insurance program appears solid, and therefore there will be continuing political pressures to make that move. The real question then appears to be when, rather than if, the United States will ever join the other advanced democracies and create a truly universal healthcare system.

Notes

Chapter 1

[1] In fairness, some of these are suicides who may well have found other means of committing the act, but guns do make it easier.

[2] This insurance may be subsidized either directly to the insured or through insurance companies.

[3] As we will discuss later (Chapter 9), some of the prescribing of additional tests is related to defensive practice by physicians as a means of protection against malpractice.

[4] Contaminated water still kills millions of people in less-developed countries, accounting in part for the very high levels of infant mortality in some countries shown in Table 1.2.

[5] This survey was funded by PHRMA, representing the pharmaceutical industry.

[6] I say "alleged" because the stem cell lines being used in most research have been in use since the administration of George W. Bush.

Chapter 2

[1] These differences are primarily because insurance is regulated at the state level so policies written in one state may not meet the specific requirements of another state.

[2] Medicare and Medicaid do monitor billings by physicians, but private health insurance companies do much less.

[3] The Centers for Medicare and Medicaid Services also inspects and approves these facilities, and certifies them as appropriate for its insured.

[4] There were so few infant deaths in Vermont that the Centers for Disease Control and Prevention did not calculate a rate.

[5] In the United States, social security eligibility is based on contributing while employed or self-employed, but Medicare is based on age alone.

[6] This reduces the administrative costs within the healthcare system, which is a significant part of total health spending in the United States.

[7] This would be analogous to the "Medigap" insurance sold in the United States to Medicare recipients (see Chapter 3).

Chapter 3

[1] That compares to less than 9 percent in 2021.

[2] Also, like Medicaid expansion contained within the Affordable Care Act, states could opt out of the program and some conservative Southern and Western states did.

[3] The states are also involved in the administration of Medicaid.

[4] The average social security check in 2023 was $1,706 per month.

[5] This amount includes the amount paid by the plan, so the insured is not out-of-pocket for the entire amount.

[6] The same skepticism exists for social security pensions, which have also been the subject of discussions about potential bankruptcy.

[7] The federal government does charge excise taxes on products such as alcohol and gasoline, but general sales taxes have been state and local revenue sources.

Chapter 4

[1] This decision is ideologically driven rather than driven by the health needs of the population, and offering contraception could almost certainly save money for the states. In 2021, over

42 percent of all births in the United States were paid for by Medicaid (National Center for Health Statistics, 2023).

2   They are called this after section 1115 of the Social Security Act, which gives the Secretary of Health and Human Services the authority to approve the waivers.

3   The premiums paid by workers for health insurance have been increasing, as employers reduce subsidies, and health prices continue to rise. See p. 100.

4   This finding may be because Democratic respondents favor a more generous program that would help low-income people even more.

Chapter 5

1   The election of 2020 produced the same pattern of control by the Democratic Party, but differences within the party—especially in the Senate—have made it difficult for President Biden to legislate effectively.

2   The most dramatic case was Senator John McCain (R-AZ), shortly before his death in 2018, dramatically making a thumbs down sign on the Senate floor ending any chance of repeal.

3   In fairness, Obama campaigned more on the principle of having some form of national health insurance than he did on the specifics of a program. This strategy was effective politically because he did not lose support from those who were wedded to one program or another.

4   Ordinarily, legislation in the Senate can be stopped by a filibuster unless there are 60 votes available to end debate. Under the reconciliation provisions of the Congressional Budget and Impoundment Control Act of 1974, legislation involving changes in revenues, expenditures and public debt cannot be stopped by a filibuster and can pass with one-half plus one votes. This was designed especially for mandatory or entitlement spending.

5   The requirement to cover contraception would be important later in the legal challenges to the law.

6   https://www.healthcare.gov/choose-a-plan/plans-categories/.

7   Some of the states use the federal computer platform but have their own programs.

8   The tax is only paid on earned income, not on income from investments, real estate, etc.; hence, even with the increases in rates for the more affluent the tax is slightly regressive. The Health Care and Education Reconciliation Act of 2010, a companion to the ACA, did impose a tax on investment income of 3.8 percent. This increased Medicare tax was estimated to have raised $10 billion in 2019, and the income tax to have raised $38 billion (Internal Revenue Service, 2022). Provisions in President Biden's budget introduced in March, 2023 would raise the tax on the more affluent and include unearned income (Tankersley and Sanger-Katz, 2023).

9   This tax was intended as much to prevent skin cancer as to raise revenue.

10   Given that the subsidies for the individual policies are delivered through the tax system, they are administered by the IRS. The need to coordinate this agency with those in the Department of Health and Human Services is but one of the many complexities involved in the ACA.

11   Some of this reluctance to cooperate also seemed to reflect a fear that the program would succeed, and would be a major achievement for a Democratic administration. That fear has taken some time to be realized, but a majority of the public do now support the program.

12   Only two counties in Alabama currently have more than one insurer.

13   567 U.S. 519 (2012).

14   If you choose to read this opinion, you will find that the logic for declaring the mandate a tax is somewhat tortured.

15   576 U.S. 473 (2015).

16   140 S.Ct. 2367(2020).

17   573 U.S. 682 (2014).

18   593 U.S. (2021).

19   In US law a party must be materially and differentially harmed in order to be able to sue. The Supreme Court said that the state government was not so harmed, and therefore there was no suit.

Chapter 6

[1] The book was as much about the need for socialism in the United States as it was about food safety, but the food safety issue was more acceptable to most politicians. The book also helped produce changes in the Meat Inspection Act.

[2] Latter-day muckraking journalists continue to be important in dealing with health issues, such as the opioid crisis and the role of Purdue Pharma in perpetuating the crisis.

[3] This was significant because it was not uncommon for cosmetics at the time to contain dangerous substances such as lead and arsenic.

[4] Thalidomide has since been shown to be a very useful drug for cancer and several infectious diseases, when used properly.

[5] Examples would be Tamoxifin, vaccines and gene therapy.

[6] Each university or medical center has an institutional review board responsible for ensuring that any testing involving human subjects is conducted in a safe and ethical manner.

[7] It was later shown that the manufacturer, Merck, had possibly manipulated some of the data used to gain approval. See Union of Concerned Scientists (2017).

[8] This study comes from a somewhat biased source, given that health insurers could charge lower rates if prescription medications were not so expensive. There is, however, other evidence that drug companies do spend extremely large amounts of money on sales and post-marketing.

[9] The best known is MRSA (Methicillin-resistant Staphylococcus Aureus).

[10] Americans spend an average of $5 per person per day for these supplements. Since many people do not use the supplements, the average expenditure for those who do is substantially higher.

[11] The Department of Housing and Urban Development was involved because the driving force behind the issuing of a certificate was the need of a local community.

[12] For a detailed analysis of the effects of certificates of need, see Conover and Bailey (2020).

[13] Some economists have argued that allowing insurance to be sold across state lines would increase competition and would therefore drive down total costs.

Chapter 7

[1] This is an estimate, and other estimates put the number substantially lower. See McDermott et al. (2020).

[2] In the states that have not expanded Medicaid coverage after the ACA the threshold for coverage under the program is higher, so more people are likely to fall into the group that is "too rich to be poor" relative to health insurance.

[3] Average income for Asian-Americans is slightly higher than for whites.

[4] I will point out in a subsequent chapter that distrust of the medical establishment also reduces the quality of healthcare provided to African-Americans.

[5] See also https://www.shepscenter.unc.edu/programs-projects/rural-health/rural-hospital-closures/.

[6] One explanation is that, in addition to lower income than in some specialities, geriatricians tend to see only patients in decline and therefore they find their jobs rather depressing.

[7] Indeed, the outcomes may be better, given the dangers of post-operative infections in hospitals (Taylor, 2016).

[8] The Community Health Aide Program in Alaska is a good example of this type of program. See https://akchap.org/.

Chapter 8

[1] The total CPI includes medical prices so if they were removed the difference would be even greater.

[2] Despite dozens of attempts, Republicans have never been able to repeal the Affordable Care Act once it had begun to create recognizable benefits for citizens.

3   There are options for bonuses and special forms of hiring in some cases, but the salaries will still be much lower than for executives in the private sector. For example, Dr Anthony Fauci, a major player in the pandemic, earns just over $400,000, as the highest paid employee in the federal government.

4   This is not just for prestige, it is also because the best doctors will attract the most patients and fill the most beds.

5   These constraints on prescribing also create complaints that they limit clinical freedom, and also may reduce quality (see Chapter 9). Physicians and their staffs may have to spend hours negotiating with low-level officials in the insurance companies in order to prescribe an expensive drug, even if it is the most appropriate.

6   This is used for extreme allergic reactions, especially to insect stings.

7   Again, this practice may affect quality because it will cause patients to request drugs that may be inappropriate for them, despite the glowing reports they see on television or in magazines.

8   For example, one study found that compensation for hospital CEOs in 2018 ranged between $274,000 and $1.4 million, and that these pay rates had almost doubled over ten years (Sullivan, 2018). Remember that many of these hospitals are non-profits, and the CEOs of large health insurance companies and pharmaceutical firms earn even more (Herman, 2021).

9   $$ICER = \frac{\text{Cost of new technology} - \text{Cost of SoC}}{\text{QALYS generated by new technology} - \text{QALYs under SoC}}$$

10   In many cases these are reimportations of American-made drugs that can be bought from Canada less expensively.

11   On pharmacy benefit managers, see Lyles (2017).

12   For example, Senate Republican leader Mitch McConnell (R-KY) called attempts to control drug prices "socialist".

13   Australia, Canada, France, Germany, Japan and the United Kingdom.

Chapter 9

1   For example, infant mortality depends on medical care, but it also depends on nutrition and on proper care for the child. Life expectancy is affected by nutrition, air and water quality, housing, and a host of other factors.

2   This phrase is at the heart of the statute that established Inspectors General in all federal agencies during the Carter administration.

3   On attitudes to Medicaid rates, see Tucker (2002).

4   This is a generic description. Some states have separate boards for doctors and nurses (and for practitioners such as physician assistants) while others combine some or all of these licensing activities.

5   In terms of quality the older medication may have more information about side-effects and hence can be used more safely.

6   Citizens are not as naive about the quality of care and the motivations of providers as they might be thought to be. See Gerber et al. (2014).

7   The law firms usually also pay for expert witnesses, depositions, etc.

8   *State Farm Mutual Automobile Insurance Co. v Campbell* 538 U.S. 408 (2003).

Chapter 10

1   As already noted (pp. 36–7) overhead costs of private insurance are approximately four to five times as high as for Medicare. There may be more overhead with these plans, but still nothing like the costs involved in managing private insurance.

2   For example, Federal Crop Insurance, insurance for banking deposits through the Federal Deposit Insurance Corporation and the Federal Savings and Loan Insurance Corporation, and Export Credit Insurance. And, of course, Medicare is an insurance program.

Notes

3   This is especially true for Senator Bernie Sanders (I-VT) who made extended health insurance perhaps the central point in his campaign for the Democratic nomination for president in 2020. He also introduced a Medicare for All bill in 2022.

4   These figures come from Gallup polls of healthcare found at: https://news.gallup.com/poll/4708/healthcare-system.aspx.

5   Historically, the CDC has been populated by bench scientists attempting to understand the nature of diseases, the mutations of viruses, etc. They were not interested in, nor very good at, explaining this work to the public but the demands are now clear that they need to do so.

References

Abbasi, K. (2020) Life, Liberty and an Independent NHS, *Journal of the Royal Society of Medicine* 1, 1–3.

Abelson, R. and M. Sanger-Katz (2023) New Medicare Rule Aims to Take Back $4.7 Billion from Insurers, *New York Times*, January 30.

Adam, C., S. Hurka, C. Knill, B.G. Peters and Y. Steinbach (2019) Introducing Vertical Policy Coordination to Comparative Policy Analysis: The Missing Link between Policy Production and Implementation, *Journal of Comparative Policy Analysis* 21, 499–517.

Adelman, R.D., M.G. Greene and M.G. Ory (2000) Communication Between Older Patients and their Physicians, *Clinics in Geriatric Medicine* 16 (February).

Alcendor, D.J. (2020) Racial Disparities-Associated COVID-19 Mortality Among Minority Populations in the US, *Journal of Clinical Medicine* 9, 2442–8.

Alderwick, H. and L.M. Gottlieb (2019) Meanings and Misunderstandings: A Social Determinants of Health Lexicon for Health Care Systems, *Milbank Quarterly* 97, 407–19.

Alford, R. (1975) *Health Care Politics: Barriers to Reform* (Chicago: University of Chicago Press).

Allen, H., B.J. Wright, K. Harding and L. Broffman (2014) The Role of Stigma in Access to Health Care for the Poor, *Milbank Fund Quarterly* 92, 289–318.

Allman, R.L. (2003) The Relationship Between Physicians and the Pharmaceutical Industry, *HEC Forum* 15, 155–204.

Altman, D. (2021) Corporate Leaders are Getting Bullish on Government Action on Health Care Costs, *KFF Perspectives,* April 29. https://www.kff.org/health-costs/perspective/corporate-leaders-are-getting-bullish-on-government-action-on-health-care-costs/?utm_campaign=KFF-2021-Drew-Columns&utm_medium=email&_hsmi=124199252&_hsenc=p2ANqtz-_h-7ttWObRN_XS0L-uBrcfPzYo_vmZMUFImAXe7P6E4_ytasvbEoBeqkg6EKbxmChU5Rtr3OcrQu7oPeZphby6CfiHIw&utm_content=124199252&utm_source=hs_email

American Association of Physician Assistants (AAPA) (2022) State Laws and Regulations. https://www.aapa.org/advocacy-central/state-advocacy/state-laws-and-regulations/

American Health Insurance Plans (AHIP) (2021) New Study Finds Big Pharma Spent More on Sales and Marketing than R&D During Pandemic, *Campaign for Sustainable Rx Pricing*, October 27. https://www.csrxp.org/icymi-new-study-finds-big-pharma-spent-more-on-sales-and-marketing-than-rd-during-pandemic/

American Hospital Association (2022) *Closure of Rural Hospitals Threatens Access to Care* (Chicago: American Hospital Association).

American Medical Association (AMA) (2022) *Residency Burnout Survey* (Chicago: AMA).

Amin, K., K. Pollitz, G. Claxton, M. Rae and C. Cox (2021) Ground Ambulance Rides and the Potential for Surprise Billing, *Peterson-KFF Health Tracker*, June 24. https://www.healthsystemtracker.org/brief/ground-ambulance-rides-and-potential-for-surprise-billing/?_hsmi=136019969&_hsenc=p2ANqtz-_m9I8EyfZKX-yh17hSV8vPoJF__j9vXshk6RvpbBgDqpkZFOsMBvBsukuTwcWBxwpemX5j8MlYBV9FVFfmf6tSMWfsbA&utm_campaign=KFF-2021-Health-Costs&utm_medium=email&utm_content=136019969&utm_source=hs_email

Angell, M. (2009) Drug Companies & Doctors: A Story of Corruption, *New York Review of Books* 56, January 15.

Bagley, N. and R. Sachs (2021) The Drug that Could Break America's Health Care, *The Atlantic*, June 11.

Barbehön, M. (2022) Policy Design and Constructivism, in B.G. Peters and G. Fontaine, eds., *Research Handbook of Policy Design* (Cheltenham: Edward Elgar).

Barrett, C.B. and J.G. McPeak (2006) Poverty Traps and Safety Nets, in A. de Janvry and R. Kanbur, eds., *Poverty, Inequality and Development Essays in Honor of Erik Thorbecke* (Heidelberg: Springer).

Barry, E. (2020) An Army of Virus Tracers Takes Place in Massachusetts, *New York Times*, April 16.

Bauchner, H., B. Fontanarosa and A.E. Thompson (2015) Professionalism, Governance and Self-Regulation of Medicine, *Journal of the American Medical Association* 313, 1831–6.

Bauder, R., T.M. Khoshgoftaer and N. Seliya (2017) A Survey of the State of Healthcare Upcoding Fraud Analysis and Detection, *Health Services and Outcomes: Research Methodology* 17, 31–55.

Beard, M. (2023) Rural Hospitals Say They Are Stuck Between a Rock and a Hard Place, *Washington Post*, January 17.

Bêland, D., P.B. Rocco and A. Walden (2019) Policy Feedback and the Politics of the Affordable Care Act, *Policy Studies Journal* 47, 395–422.

Belluck, P. (2021) FDA Will Permanently Allow Abortion Pills by Mail, *New York Times*, December 16.

Besser, R.E. (2020) We Can't Allow the CDC to be Tainted by Politics, *Scientific American*, September 15. https://www.scientificamerican.com/article/we-cant-allow-the-cdc-to-be-tainted-by-politics/?gclid=Cj0KCQjw3eeXBhD7ARIsAHjssr8cVlkV5WEJX20kXgzPNz9EQ_NuwioSuGZnWHLK2p-x4GAj_6OugOYaAiPKEALw_wcB

Best, M.J., E.G. McFarland, G.F. Anderson and U. Srikumarian (2020) The Likely Economic Effect of Fewer Elective Surgical Procedures on US Hospitals During the COVID-19 Pandemic, *Surgery* 168, 962–7.

Blake, A. (2020) Trump Finds Someone to Blame for Corona Virus: Andrew Cuomo, *Washington Post*, March 24.

Blumberg, L.J., J. Holahan, S. McMorrow and M. Simpson (2020) *Estimating the Impact of a Public Option or Capping Provider Payment Rates* (Washington, DC: Urban Institute).

Booth, S. (2019) Up to 80% of Hospital Bills Have Errors: Are You Being Overcharged? *Healthline*, May 21. https://www.healthline.com/health-news/80-percent-hospital-bills-have-errors-are-you-being-overcharged

Born, P.H., J.B. Karl and W.K. Viscusi (2017) The Net Effects of Medical Malpractice Tort Reform on Health Insurance Losses: The Texas Experience, *Health Economics Review* 7. https://doi.org/10.1186/s13561-017-0174-2

Botting, J. (2002) The History of Thalidomide, *Drug News & Perspectives*, November 1. https://europepmc.org/article/med/12677202

Bovbjerg, R.R., L.C. Dubay, G.M. Kenney and S.A. Norton (1996) Defensive Medicine and Tort Reform: New Evidence in Old Bottles, *Journal of Health Politics, Policy and Law* 21, 267–88.

Boyle, P. (2021) Medical School Applicants and Enrollments Reach Record Highs, *AAMCNEWS*, December 8. https://www.aamc.org/news-insights/medical-school-applicants-and-enrollments-hit-record-highs-underrepresented-minorities-lead-surge

Brinker, L. (2014) Vermont Abandons Plan for Single Payer Health Care, *Salon*, December 18. https://www.salon.com/2014/12/18/vermont_abandons_plan_for_single_payer_health_care/

British Medical Association (BMA) (2022) NHS Backlog Data Analysis, August 15. https://www.bma.org.uk/advice-and-support/nhs-delivery-and-workforce/pressures/nhs-backlog-data-analysis

Brodie, M., E.C. Hamel and M. Norton (2015) Medicare as Reflected in Public Opinion, *Generations: Journal of the American Society on Aging* 39, 134–41.

Burwell, S.M. (2015) Setting Value-based Payment Goals–HHS Efforts to Improve U.S. Health Care, *New England Journal of Medicine* 372, 897–99.

Cahn, Z. and E.M. Johnston (2018) Clintoncare and Obamacare: Lessons from Gridlock Theory, *Congress & the Presidency* 45, 225–53.

Callahan, D. (2009) *Taming the Beloved Beast: How Medical Technology Costs are Destroying Our Health Care System* (Princeton, NJ: Princeton University Press).

Cameron, K.A., J. Song, L.M. Manheim and D.D. Dunlop (2010) Gender Disparities in Health and Healthcare Use Among Older Adults, *Journal of Women's Health* 19, 1643–50.

Campbell, E.C. (2007) Doctors and Drug Companies—Scrutinizing Influential Relations, *New England Journal of Medicine* 357, 1796–7.

Capano, G., A.R. Zito, F. Toth and J. Rayner (2022) *Trajectories of Governance: How States Shaped Policy Sectors in the Neoliberal Age* (London: Macmillan).

Capretta, J.C. (2020) Washington State's Quasi-Public Option, *Milbank Quarterly* 98, 14–17.

Carpenter, D.P. (2010) *Reputation and Power: Organizational Image and Pharmaceutical Regulation at the FDA* (Princeton, NJ: Princeton University Press).

Carroll, A.E. (2022) What's Wrong with Health Insurance? Deductibles are Ridiculous for a Start, *New York Times*, July 7.

Center for Medicare and Medicaid Studies (2022) *Age Distribution of Healthcare Costs* (Washington, DC: Department of Health and Human Services).

Centers for Medicare and Medicaid Services (CMS) (2020) *2020 Estimated Improper Payment Rates for Centers for Medicare and Medicaid (CMS) Programs* (Washington, DC: CMS).

Chaikind, H. (2010) *Individual Mandate and Related Information Requirement under PPACA* (Washington, DC: Congressional Research Service).

Chassin, M.R. and J.M. Loeb (2013) High-Reliability Health Care: Getting from Here to There, *Milbank Quarterly* 91, 459–90.

Clemens, J., B.N. Ippolito and S. Veuger (2021) Medicaid and Fiscal Federalism During the COVID-19 Pandemic, *NBER Working Paper 28670* (Cambridge, MA: National Bureau of Economic Research).

CNN (2009) Senate Panel Votes Down Public Option for Health Care Bill, *CNN*, September 29. https://edition.cnn.com/2009/POLITICS/09/29/senate.public.option/

Cohen, J. (2021) Insulin's Out of Pocket Cost Burden to Diabetic Patients Continues to Rise, *Forbes*, January 5. https://www.forbes.com/sites/joshuacohen/2021/01/05/insulins-out-of-pocket-cost-burden-to-diabetic-patients-continues-to-rise-despite-reduced-net-costs-to-pbms/?sh=1371ade040b2

Cohn, J. (2021) *The Ten Year War: Obamacare and the Unfinished Crusade for Universal Coverage* (New York: St. Martin's).

Colander, D. (2017) Reforming the Affordable Care Act, *Eastern Economic Journal* 43, 173–9.

Collins, S.R., M.Z. Gunja and G.N. Aboulafia (2020) U.S. Health Insurance Coverage in 2020: A Looming Crisis in Affordability, *Commonwealth Fund Issue Brief*, August 19.

Collins, S.R., M.Z. Gunja and M.M. Doty (2017) How Well Does Insurance Coverage Protect Consumers from Health Care Costs, Commonwealth Fund, *Issue Brief*, October. https://www.commonwealthfund.org/sites/default/files/documents/___media_files_publications_issue_brief_2017_oct_collins_underinsured_biennial_ib.pdf

Commonwealth Fund (2022a) *Meeting America's Public Health Challenge* (New York: Commonwealth Fund).

Commonwealth Fund (2022b) *The State of U.S. Health Insurance in 2022* (New York: Commonwealth Fund).

Congressional Budget Office (CBO) (2016) *Federal Subsidies for Health Insurance Coverage for People Under Age 65: 2016 to 2026* (Washington, DC: CBO).

Congressional Budget Office (CBO) (2020) *Who Went Without Health Insurance in 2019?* (Washington, DC: CBO).

Conover, C.J. and J. Bailey (2020) Certificate of Need Laws: A Systematic Review and Cost-Effectiveness Analysis, *BMC Health Services Research* 20. https://doi.org/10.1186/s12913-020-05563-1

Corbie-Smith, G. (1999) The Continuing Legacy of the Tuskegee Syphilis Study: Considerations for Clinical Investigation, *American Journal of Medical Science* 317, 5–8.

Cox, C., K. Amin and J. Ortaliza (2022) Five Things to Know About the Possible Renewal of Extra Affordable Care Act Subsidies, *Kaiser Family Foundation*, July 22. https://www.kff.org/policy-watch/five-things-to-know-about-possible-renewal-of-extra-affordable-care-act-subsidies/

Cubanski, J., T. Neuman and M. Freed (2023) Explaining the Prescription Drug Provisions in the Inflation Reduction Act, *KFF Medicare*, January 24. https://www.kff.org/medicare/issue-brief/explaining-the-prescription-drug-provisions-in-the-inflation-reduction-act/

Davies, E.H., E. Fulton, D. Brook and D.A. Hughes (2017) Affordable Orphan Drugs: A Role for Not-for-Profit Organizations, *British Journal of Clinical Pharmacology* 83, 1595–601.

Davis, K. and C. Schoen (1978) *Health and the War on Poverty: A Ten-Year Appraisal* (Washington, DC: The Brookings Institution).

Davis, S. (2009) Palin's "Death Panels" Charge Named "Lie of the Year". *The Wall Street Journal*, December 22.

Daw, J.R., E. Eckert, H.L. Allen and K. Underhill (2021) Extending Postpartum Medicaid: State and Federal Policy Options During and After COVID-19, *Journal of Health Politics, Policy and Law* 46, 505–26.

de Bienassis, K., S. Kristensen, M. Burtscher, I. Brownwood and N.S. Klazinga (2020) *Culture as a Cure: Assessments of Patient Safety Cultures in OECD Countries*, OECD Health Working Paper 119 (Paris: OECD).

DeBonis, M. (2016) Obama Vetoes Republican Repeal of Health-care Law, *Washington Post*, January 8.

Dickman, S.L., D.U. Himmelstein and S. Woolhandler (2017) Inequality and the Health-care System in the United States, *The Lancet* 389, 1431–41.

Donnelly, K.P. and D.A. Rochefort (2012) The Lessons of "Lesson Drawing": How the Obama Administration Attempted to Learn from the Failure of the Clinton Health Plan, *Journal of Policy History* 24, 184–233.

Doty, M.M., R. Tikkanen, A. Shah and E.C. Schneider (2020) Primary Care Physicians' Role in Coordinating Medical and Health-Related Social Needs in Eleven Countries, *Health Affairs* 39, 115–23.

Dovido, J.F., S. Eggly, T.L. Albrecht, N. Hagiwara and L.A. Penner (2016) Racial Bias in Medicine and Healthcare Disparities, *TPM* 23, 489–510.

Dranove, D., C. Ody and A. Stare (2017) *A Dose of Managed Care: Controlling Drug Spending in Medicaid*, NBER Working Paper 23956 (October).

Draper, R. (2019) How "Medicare for All" Went Mainstream, *New York Times Magazine*, August 27.

Ebeler, J., T. Neuman, and J. Cubanski (2011) The Independent Payment Advisory Board: A New Approach to Controlling Medicare Spending, *Kaiser Family Foundation*, April 13.

Ehrenreich, B. (2018) *Natural Causes: An Epidemic of Wellness, The Certainty of Dying, and Killing Ourselves to Live Longer* (New York: Twelve).

Elg, M., B. Kollberg and K. Palmberg (2013) Performance Measurement to Drive Improvements in Healthcare Practice, *International Journal of Operations & Production Management* 33, 1623–51.

Emerson, J. (2022) Hospitals that See Most Black Patients Are Paid Less than Other Hospitals, Report Says, *Becker's Hospital Review*, August 4. https://www.beckershospitalreview.com/health-equity/hospitals-that-see-the-most-black-patients-are-paid-less-than-other-hospitals-report-finds.html?origin=BHRE&utm_source=BHRE&utm_medium=email&utm_content=newsletter&oly_enc_id=6522A1601390C5Z

Enthoven, A. (1994) Why Not the Clinton Health Plan?, *Inquiry* 31, 129–35.

Ess, S.M., S. Schneeweiss and T.D. Szucs (2003) European Healthcare Policies for Controlling Drug Expenditures, *Pharmacoeconomica* 2, 89–103.

Falkson, S.R. and V.N. Srinivasan (2022) Health Maintenance Organizations, *Stats Pearl*, March 9. https://www.ncbi.nlm.nih.gov/books/NBK554454/

Feder, J.M. (1977) *Medicare: The Politics of Federal Hospital Insurance* (Lanham, MD; Lexington Books).

Feldman, R. (2022) We Need a Labeling System for Pharmaceutical Prices, *Washington Post*, June 10.

Fields, D., E. Leshen and K. Patel (2010) Driving Quality Gains and Cost Savings Through Adoption of Medical Homes, *Health Affairs* 29, 819–26.

Fisher, J.A. (2007) "Ready to Recruit" or "Ready to Consent" Populations? Informed Consent and the Limits of Subject Autonomy, *Qualitative Inquiry* 13, 875–94.

Florko, N. and E. Welle (2022) The FDA Stands by as the Vaping Industry Flouts its Orders, *STATNEWS*, August 24. https://www.statnews.com/2022/08/24/the-fda-stands-by-as-the-vaping-industry-flouts-its-orders/

Frakt, A.B., S.D. Pizer, and R. Feldman (2011) Should Medicare Adopt the Veterans Health Administration Formulary?, *Health Economics* 21, 485–95.

Frankenfield, J. (2020) Which Industry Spends Most on Lobbying?, *Investopedia*, May 7. https://www.investopedia.com/investing/which-industry-spends-most-lobbying-antm-so/

Fraser, M. (2013) The Affordable Care Attack, *New Labor Forum* 20, 96–8.

Frates, C. and C.B. Brown (2009) Gang of Six Could Hold Obama's Fate, *Politico*, September 8.

Freed, M., J.F. Biniek, A. Damico and T. Neuman (2022) Medicare Advantage in 2022: Enrollment Update and Key Trends, *Kaiser Family Foundation*, August 25. https://www.kff.org/medicare/issue-brief/medicare-advantage-in-2022-enrollment-update-and-key-trends/?utm_campaign=KFF-2022-The-Latest&utm_medium=email&_hsmi=224105895&_hsenc=p2ANqtz-_un-a05W5wKqXGY04G7Dl6Kt6wZXmD6ZqyFq0gDakvGHJYEgAqHsJ4b3R8hb0b0K_uSFoAVvJjSi6R5pYU1TXO5VB7Cw&utm_content=224105895&utm_source=hs_email

References

Fronstin, P. and S.A. Woodbury (2020) How Many Americans Have Lost Jobs with Employer Health Coverage During the Pandemic?, *Commonwealth Fund Issue Brief*, October 7. https://www.commonwealthfund.org/publications/issue-briefs/2020/oct/how-many-lost-jobs-employer-coverage-pandemic

Frosch, D.L., D. Grande, D.M. Tarn and R.L. Kravitz (2010) A Decade of Controversy: Balancing Policy with Evidence in the Regulation of Prescription Drug Advertising, *American Journal of Public Health* 100, 24–32.

Furlow, B. (2019) Skepticism about new US Government Hospital Pricing Transparency Rule, *Lancet Oncology* 20, 188.

Gamble, M. (2021) Stop Assuming Black Americans Don't Want the Vaccine because of Tuskegee, Critics Say, *Becker Hospital Report*, March 24. https://www.beckershospitalreview.com/public-health/stop-assuming-black-americans-don-t-want-the-vaccine-because-of-tuskegee-critics-say.html?origin=BHRE&utm_source=BHRE&utm_medium=email&utm_content=newsletter&oly_enc_id=6522A1601390C5Z

Garrison, L.P. and A. Towse (2017) Value-based Pricing and Reimbursement in Personalized Healthcare: An Introduction to the Basic Health Economics, *Journal of Personalized Medicine* 7. http://dx.doi.org/10.3390/jpm7030010

GE Healthcare (2019) How Much Does an MRI Cost? https://www.gehealthcare.com/feature-article/how-much-does-an-mri-cost?utm_medium=cpc&utm_source=google&utm_campaign=USC-PS-2021-REG-AlwaysOn&utm_term=&utm_content=12518725892&npclid=Cj0KCQjw16KFBhCgARIsALB0g8IyOBkdvPvwl62QrWNuPGqz2-NQ4MzoypTe-3ltAnWkI5cbnglAANEaAi1_EALw_wcB&gclid=Cj0KCQjw16KFBhCgARIsALB0g8IyOBkdvPvwl62QrWNuPGqz2-NQ4MzoypTe-3ltAnWkI5cbnglAANEaAi1_EALw_wcB

Gellad, W.F., S. Schneeweiss, P. Beawarsky, S. Lipsitz and J.S. Haas (2008) What if the Federal Government Negotiated Pharmaceutical Prices for Seniors? An Estimate of National Savings, *Journal of General Internal Medicine* 23, 1435–40.

Gerber, A.S., E.M. Patashnik, D. Doherty and C.M. Dowling (2014) Doctors Know Best: Physician Endorsements, Public Opinion and the Politics of Comparative Effectivness Research, *Journal of Health Politics, Policy and Law* 39, 171–208.

Giaimo, S. (2009) *Markets and Medicine: The Politics of Health Care Reform in Britain, Germany and the United States* (Ann Arbor: University of Michigan Press).

Giaquinto, A.N., K.D. Miller, K.V. Tossas, R.A. Winn, A. Jemal and R.L. Siegel (2022) Cancer Statistics for African-American/Black People, CA, *A Cancer Journal for Clinicians* 72, 209–33.

Girvan, G. and A. Roy (2020) United States: #4 in World Index of Medical Innovation, *freopp.org.* https://freopp.org/united-states-health-system-profile-4-in-the-world-index-of-healthcare-innovation-b593ba15a96

Gold, J. and S. Kliff (2018) A Baby was Treated with a Nap and a Bottle of Formula. The Bill was $18,000, *Kaiser Health Network*, July 2.

Gold, M., M. Sparer and K. Chu (1996) Marketwatch: Medicaid Managed Care: Lessons from Five States, *Health Affairs* 15, 153–66.

Goldacre, B. (2014) *Bad Pharma: How Drug Companies Mislead Doctors and Harm Patients* (New York: Parrar, Strauss and Giroux).

Gonzalez, O. (2023) FDA adds a Major New Twist to Abortion Pill Fight, *Axios*, January 4. https://www.axios.com/newsletters/axios-vitals-56516afa-ae85-4bbb-9558-135a255376c0.html?chunk=0&utm_term=emshare#story0

Gooch, K. (2016) Medical Billing Errors Growing, Says Medical Billing Advocates of America, *Becker's Hospital Review*, April 12. https://www.beckershospitalreview.com/finance/medical-billing-errors-growing-says-medical-billing-advocates-of-america.html

Gordon, S.H., N. Huberfeld and D.K. Jones (2020) What Federalism Means for US Response to Coronavirus Disease, *Journal of the American Medical Association*, Health Forum, May 8.

Gostin, L.O. and S. Nass (2009) Reforming the HIPAA Privacy Rule: Safeguarding Privacy and Promoting Research, *Journal of the American Medical Association* 301, 1373–5.

Govindarajan, R., H. Kaur and A. Yelam (2019) Understanding System Errors, in R. Govindarajan, H. Kaur and A. Yelam, eds., *Improving Patient Safety* (New York: Productivity Press).

Greene, J., J. Blustein and B.C. Weitzman (2006) Race, Segregation and Physicians' Participation in Medicaid, *Milbank Quarterly* 84, 239–72.

Greep, N.C., S. Woolhandler and D. Himmelstein (2021) Physician Burnout: Fix the Doctor or Fix the System, *American Journal of Medicine* 135, 416–17.

Greer, S.L. (2016) Devolution and Health in the UK: Policy and Its Lessons since 1998, *British Medical Bulletin* 118, 16–24.

Griffith, K., D.K. Jones and B.D. Sommers (2018) Diminishing Insurance Choices in Affordable Care Act Marketplaces: A County-based Analysis, *Health Affairs* 37, 1678–84.

Grimm, C.A. (2022) *Some Medicare Advantage Organizations Denials of Prior Authorization Requests Raise Concerns About Beneficiary Access to Medically Necessary Care* (Washington, DC: Office of the Inspector General, Department of Health and Human Services), April.

Gudiksen, K.L. and J.S. King (2019) The Burden of Federalism: Challenges to State Attempts at Controlling Prescription Drug Costs, *Journal of Legal Medicine* 39, 95–120.

Haeder, S.F. and D.L. Weimer (2013) You Can't Make Me Do It: State Implementation of Insurance Exchanges under the Affordable Care Act, *Public Administration Review* 73, 534–47.

Haefner, M. (2021) Biden Zeroes in on Healthcare Competition in Executive Order, *Becker's Hospital Review*, July 9. https://www.beckershospitalreview.com/hospital-management-administration/biden-zeros-in-on-healthcare-competition-in-executive-order-10-notes.html

Ham, C. (2020) *Health Policy in Britain: The Politics and Organization of the National Health Service* (London: Routledge).

Hamel, L., C. Muñana and M. Brodie (2019) Kaiser Family Foundation/LA Times Survey of Adults with Employer-Sponsored Health Insurance, *Kaiser Family Foundation*, May. https://files.kff.org/attachment/Report-KFF-LA-Times-Survey-of-Adults-with-Employer-Sponsored-Health-Insurance

References

Hart, W. (2022) CVS's Latest Moves to Expand Primary Care and Health Insurance Offerings, *Benefits Pro*, August 11. https://www.benefitspro.com/2022/08/11/cvss-latest-moves-to-expand-primary-care-and-health-insurance-offerings/?slreturn=20220714143926

Healy, M. (2022) As Global Health Threats Evolved, the CDC Didn't, *Los Angeles Times*, August 20.

Henry, T.A. (2021) Why 41% of Patients Have Skipped Care During the COVID-19 Pandemic, *AMA: Public Health*, February 15. https://www.ama-assn.org/delivering-care/public-health/why-41-patients-have-skipped-care-during-covid-19-pandemic

Herd, P., T. DeLeire, H. Harvey and D.P. Moynihan (2013) Shifting Administrative Burden to the State: The Case of Medicaid Take-up, *Public Administration Review* 73, S69–81.

Herman, B. (2021) Health Care Executive Pay Soars During Pandemic, *AXIOS*, June 14. https://www.axios.com/2021/06/14/health-care-ceo-pay-2020-pandemic

Hicks, J.L. and P.D. Biddinger (2020) Novel Coronavirus and Old Lessons–Preparing the Health System for the Pandemic, *New England Journal of Medicine* 382, March 25.

Himmelstein, D.U., T. Campbell and S. Woolhandler (2020) Health Care Administrative Costs in the United States and Canada, *Annals of Internal Medicine*, January 7. https://hca-mn.org/wp-content/uploads/2020/01/Adm-Costs-2017.pdf

Himmelstein, D.U., R.M. Lawless, D. Thorne, P. Foohey and S. Woolhandler (2019) Medical Bankruptcy Still Common Despite the Affordable Care Act, *American Journal of Public Health* 109, 431–3.

Hollowell, A. (2023) As Birth Rates Increase, OB-GYN Shortage Worsens, *Becker's Hospital Review*, March 17.

Howard, C. (2006) *The Welfare State Nobody Knows* (Princeton, NJ: Princeton University Press).

Iglehart, J.K. (2007) The Battle over SCHIP, *The New England Journal of Medicine* 357(10), 957–60.

Illich, I. (1975) *Medical Nemesis: The Expropriation of Health* (New York: Pantheon).

Internal Revenue Service (2022) *Questions and Answers for the Additional Medicare Tax* (Washington, DC: IRS). https://www.irs.gov/businesses/small-businesses-self-employed/questions-and-answers-for-the-additional-medicare-tax

Jacobs, L., T. Marmor and J. Oberlander (1999) The Oregon Health Plan and the Political Paradox of Rationing: What Advocates and Critics Have Claimed and What Oregon Did, *Journal of Health Politics, Policy and Law* 24,161–80.

Jacobs, L.R., S. Mettler and L. Zhu (2019) Affordable Care Act Moving to New Stage of Public Acceptance, *Journal of Health Politics, Policy and Law* 44, 911–17.

Jost, T.S. (2017) The Tax Bill and the Individual Mandate: What Happened, and What Does it Mean, *Health Affairs*. https://www.healthaffairs.org/do/10.1377/forefront.20171220.323429/full/

Jost, T.S. (2022) A Fix for the Family Glitch, *The Commonwealth Fund*, April 12, https://www.commonwealthfund.org/blog/2022/fix-family-glitch

Junewicz, A. and S.J. Youngner (2015) *Patient Care Satisfaction Surveys on a Scale of 0 to 10: Improving Health Care, or Leading it Astray?*, Hastings Center Report 45 (Garrison, NY: Hastings Center).

Kack, A. (2023) Hospital Price Transparency: Fines or Full Compliance, *Modern Healthcare*, January 24. https://www.modernhealthcare.com/finance/hospital-price-transparency-compliance-cms-deaconess-sanford

Kagan, R.A. (2003) *Adversarial Legalism: The American Way of Law* (Cambridge, MA: Harvard University Press).

Kaiser Family Foundation (KFF) (2011) *Reaching for the Stars: Quality Ratings of Medicare Advantage Plans.* www.kff.org/medicare/upload/8151.pdf

Kaiser Family Foundation (KFF) (2019) Coverage of Breast Cancer Screening and Prevention Services, *KFF Women's Health Policy*, September 26. https://www.kff.org/womens-health-policy/fact-sheet/coverage-of-breast-cancer-screening-and-prevention-services/

Kaiser Family Foundation (KFF) (2022a) Medicaid Postpartum Extension Tracker, July 13. https://www.kff.org/medicaid/issue-brief/medicaid-postpartum-coverage-extension-tracker/

Kaiser Family Foundation (KFF) (2022b) State Profiles Highlight Variations in How Many Low-income Medicare Beneficiaries Get Additional Help with Their Medicare Cases, *KFF Newsroom*, April 20.

Kapstan, R. (2011) Older Americans, Medicare and the Affordable Care Act: What's Really in It for Elders, *Generations* 1, 19–25.

Keane, M. and O. Stavrunova (2016) Adverse Selection, Moral Hazard and the Demand for Medigap Insurance, *Journal of Econometrics* 190, 62–78.

Keen, J.D. and J.E. Keen (2009) What is the Point: Will Screening Mammography Save my Life?, *BMC Medical Information Decisionmaking* 2, 9–19.

Keith, K. (2022) Biden Administration Proposes to Fix Family Glitch, *Health Affairs*, April 6. https://www.healthaffairs.org/do/10.1377/forefront.20220405.571745/

Keith, K., J. Hoardley and K. Lucia (2022) New No Surprises Act Guidance Builds on Recent Final Rule, *Health Affairs Forefront*, August 22. https://www.healthaffairs.org/do/10.1377/forefront.20220822.101536

Kelman, B. (2022) They Lost Medicaid When Paperwork was Sent to a Pasture, Signalling the Mess to Come, *NPR*, August 2. https://www.npr.org/sections/health-shots/2022/08/02/1114857641/lost-medicaid-paperwork

Kern, L.M., M. Rajan, H.A. Pincus, L.P. Casalino and S.S. Stuard (2020) Health Care Fragmentation in Medicaid Managed Care vs. Fee for Service, *Population Health Management* 23, 53–8.

Kesselheim, A.S., T.J. Hwang and J. Avon (2021) Paying for Prescription Drugs in the New Administration, *JAMA* 325, 819–20.

Khazan, O. (2021) What Americans Don't Know About Their Medications, *The Atlantic*, February 18.

Kifmann, M. (2017) Competition Policy for Health Care Provision in Germany, *Health Policy* 121, 119–25.

King, K.M. (2014) Medicare Fraud: Progress Made, But More Action Needed to Address Medicare Fraud, Waste, and Abuse, *GAO*. http://www.gao.gov/products/GAO-14-560T

Kingdon, J.W. (2003) *Agendas, Alternatives and Public Policy*, 2nd edition (Boston: Little, Brown).

Kirzinger, A., A. Kearney, M. Stokes and M. Brodie (2021) KFF Tracking Poll, May. https://www.kff.org/health-costs/poll-finding/kff-health-tracking-poll-may-2021/

Kitchen, H., M. McMillan and A. Shah (2019) *Local Public Finance and Economics* (Cham: Palgrave Macmillan). https://doi.org/10.1007/978-3-030-21986-4_11

Klein, R. (1999) Markets, Politicians, and the NHS, *British Medical Journal* 319, 1383–4.

Klein, R. (2019) *The New Politics of the NHS: From Creation to Reinvention*, 7th edition (Boca Raton, FL: CRC Press).

Kliff, S. (2013) Will Obamacare lead to Millions More Part-time Workers? Companies are Still Deciding, *Washington Post*, Wonkblog, May 6. https://web.archive.org/web/20130507073246/http://www.washingtonpost.com/blogs/wonkblog/wp/2013/05/06/will-obamacare-lead-to-millions-more-part-time-workers-companies-are-still-deciding/

Kliff, S. (2016) Why Obamacare Enrollees Voted for Trump, *Vox*, December 13. https://www.vox.com/science-and-health/2016/12/13/13848794/kentucky-obamacare-trumplost

Konrad, T.R. et al. (2010) It's About Time: Physicians' Perceptions of Time Constraints in Primary Care Practice in Three National Healthcare Systems, *Medical Care* 48, 95–100.

Krause, P.R. and M.F. Gruber (2020) Emergency Use Authorization of COVID Vaccines–Safety and Efficacy Follow-up Considerations, *New England Journal of Medicine* 383, November 5. https://www.nejm.org/doi/full/10.1056/NEJMp2031373

Kurani, N., D. Collier and C. Cox (2022) How Prescription Drug Costs in the United States Differ from other Countries, *KFF Health Systems Tracker*, February 8.

Kurani, N., G. Ramirez, I. Hudman, C. Cox and R. Kamal (2021a) Early Results from Federal Price Transparency Rule Show Difficulty in Estimating Cost of Care, Peterson, *KFF Health System Tracker*, April 9.

Kurani, N., A. Kearney, A. Kirzinger and C. Cox (2021b) Few Adults are Aware of Hospital Price Transparency Requirements, Peterson, *KFF Health System Tracker*, June 28.

LaFraniere, S. and N. Weiland (2022) Failings of CDC Prompt a Rebuke and an Overhaul, *New York Times*, August 18.

LaFraniere, S. and N. Weiland (2023) US Plans to End Public Health Emergency for COVID in May, *New York Times*, January 30.

Lalani, H.S., A.S. Kesselheim and B.N. Rome (2022) Potential Medicare Part D Savings on Generic Drugs from the Mark Cuban Cost Plus Drug Company, *Annals of Internal Medicine*, June 21. https://www.acpjournals.org/doi/10.7326/M22-0756

LaPointe, J. (2016) How the Affordable Care Act Impacted Healthcare Revenue Cycle, *Recycle Intelligence*, August 18. https://revcycleintelligence.com/news/how-the-affordable-care-act-impacted-healthcare-revenue-cycle

Lawrence, E. (2020) Nearly Half of Americans Delayed Medical Care Due to Pandemic, *Kaiser Health Network*, May 27. https://khn.org/news/nearly-half-of-americans-delayed-medical-care-due-to-pandemic/

Lawrence, M.B. (2021) Medicare "Bankruptcy", *Boston College Law Review* 63(2). https://ssrn.com/abstract=3917021 or http://dx.doi.org/10.2139/ssrn.3917021

Leonhardt, D. (2009) Limits to a System That's Sick, *New York Times*, June 17.

Leslie, C.M. (1976) *Asian Medical Systems: A Comparative Study* (Berkeley: University of California Press).

Levey, N.N. (2022) In America, Cancer Patients Endure Debt on Top of Disease, *Kaiser Health Network*, July 9. https://khn.org/news/article/in-america-cancer-patients-endure-debt-on-top-of-disease/

Levitan, S.A. and R. Taggart (1976) The Great Society Did Succeed, *Political Science Quarterly* 91, 601–18.

Lewis, T. (2022) U.S. Monkeypox Response has been Woefully Inadequate, Experts Say, *Scientific American*, July 13. https://www.scientificamerican.com/article/monkeypox-testing-and-vaccination-in-u-s-have-been-vastly-inadequate-experts-say1/?amp=true&gclid=Cj0KCQjwjIKYBhC6ARIsAGEds-J1lIkwTnnyGRly6zS5gMETmaXaweZkdoX3snjFcwoH-DPIrNBFYlUaAuVbEALw_wcB

Leys, T. (2023) They Could Lose the House—to Medicaid, *NPR News*, March 1. https://www.npr.org/sections/health-shots/2023/03/01/1159490515/they-could-lose-the-house-to-medicaid?utm_source=newsletter&utm_medium=email&utm_campaign=newsletter_axiosvitals&stream=top

Lillie-Blanton, M. and C. Hoffman (2005) The Role of Health Insurance Coverage in Reducing Racial/Ethnic Disparities in Health Care, *Health Affairs* 24. https://www.healthaffairs.org/doi/abs/10.1377/hlthaff.24.2.398

Long, S.H. and T.M. Smeeding (1984) Alternative Medicare Funding Sources, *Milbank Memorial Fund Quarterly* 62, 326–48.

Lopez, E., T. Neumang, G. Jacobsen and L. Levitt (2020) How Much More than Medicare do Private Insurers Pay? A Review of the Literature, *KFF Issue Brief*, April 15. https://www.kff.org/medicare/issue-brief/how-much-more-than-medicare-do-private-insurers-pay-a-review-of-the-literature/

Lyles, A. (2017) Pharmacy Benefit Management Companies: Do They Create Value in the US Healthcare System, *PharmoEconomics* 35, 493–500.

Lyon, J. (2016) Significant Increases in EpiPen Prices, *Journal of the American Medical Association* 316, 1439.

Lyons, B. and D. Rowland (2022) Improving Help at Home: Medicare Beneficiaries' and Caregivers' Experiences, *The Commonwealth Fund*, July 11. https://www.commonwealthfund.org/blog/2022/improving-help-home-medicare-beneficiaries-and-caregivers-experiences

Maas, S. (2022) A Dizzying Tour of Medicare's Drug Pricing Labyrinth, *Washington Post*, August 5.

Macy, E. (2020) Addressing the Epidemic of Antibiotic "Allergy" Over-diagnosis, *Annals of Allergy, Asthma and Immunology* 124, 550–7.

Mankiw, N.G. (2009) The Pitfalls of the Public Option, *New York Times*, June 28.

Mankiw, N.G. (2017) Why Health Care Policy is So Hard, *New York Times*, July 28.

Mann, C., J. Guyer, A. Striar and D. Stone (2020) The Fiscal Impact of the Trump Administration's Medicaid Block Grant Initiative, *The Commonwealth Fund*, March 6.

Marmor, T.R. (2000) *The Politics of Medicare*, 2nd edition (New York: Aldine de Gruyter).

Maruthappu, M., R. Olugunde and A. Gunarajasingam (2013) Is Health Care a Right or a Privilege? Health Reforms in the USA and their Impact Upon the Concept of Care, *Annals of Medicine and Surgery* 2, 15–17.

Matsa, D.A. and A.R. Miller (2019) Who Votes for Medicaid Expansion? Lessons from Maine's 2017 Referendum, *Journal of Health Politics, Policy and Law* 44, 563–88.

Mazer, B. and C. Nabhan (2019) No. Medical Errors Are Not the Third Leading Cause of Death, Medscape, October 6. https://www.medscape.com/viewarti cle/917696#vp_2

McDermott, D. and C. Cox (2020) Insurer Participation in ACA Marketplaces, 2014–21, *KFF*, November 23. https://www.kff.org/private-insurance/issue-brief/insurer-participation-on-the-aca-marketplaces-2014-2021/

McDermott, D., C. Cox, R. Rudowitz and R. Garfield (2020) How Has the Pandemic Affected Health Coverage in the U.S.?, *Kaiser Family Foundation Policy Watch*, December 9. https://www.kff.org/policy-watch/how-has-the-pande mic-affected-health-coverage-in-the-u-s/

McDonough, J.E. (2015) The Demise of Vermont's Single-payer Plan, *New England Journal of Medicine* 372, 1584–5.

McGuire, M.F. (2013) International Accreditation of Ambulatory Centers and Medical Tourism, *Clinics in Plastic Surgery* 40, 493–8.

McGuire, T.J., J.P. Newhouse and A.D. Sinaiko (2011) An Economic History of Medicare Part C. *Milbank Quarterly* 89, 289–332.

Medina, E. (2022) Ex-Nurse Convicted in Fatal Medication Error Gets Probation, *New York Times*, May 15.

Mensik, H. (2022) Third of Nurses Plan to Quit Their Jobs by End of 2022, Survey Shows, *Healthcaredive*, March 16. https://www.healthcaredive.com/news/ nurse-burnout-covid-quit-travel-incredible-health/620488/

Miller, E.A. (2014) *Block Granting Medicaid: A Model for 21st Century Health Reform?* (New York: Routledge, Taylor & Francis).

Minemyer, P. (2018) Hospitals Spend Big Bucks on Advertising: Here's a Look at the Cost of 8 Ad Campaigns, *Fierce Healthcare*, August 27. https://www.fierc ehealthcare.com/hospitals-health-systems/hospitals-spending-big-bucks-advertis ing-a-look-cost-8-ad-campaigns

Moore, W.J. and R.J. Newman (1993) Drug Formulary Restrictions as a Cost Containment Policy in Medicaid Programs, *Journal of Law and Economics* 36, 71–84.

Mucio, D. (2022) CMS Threatens to Ax UNC Health's Medicare Funding After Flagship Hospital Cited for Serious Noncompliance, *Fierce Healthcare*, July 13.

Mulcahy, A.W., C. Whaley, M.G. Tebeka, D. Schwam, N, Ederfield and A.U. Becerra-Ornelas (2021) *International Prescription Drug Price Comparisons: Current Empirical Estimates and Comparisons with Previous Studies* (Santa Monica, CA: Rand Corporation).

Mullin, R. (2022) California Governor Says the State Will Make its Own Insulin, *Chemical and Engineering News*, July 11. https://cen.acs.org/pharmaceuticals/California-governor-says-state-make/100/web/2022/07

National Academies of Sciences, Engineering, and Medicine (2022) *Improving Representation in Clinical Trials and Research: Building Research Equity for Women and Underrepresented Groups* (Washington, DC: The National Academies Press). https://doi.org/10.17226/26479

National Conference of State Legislatures (NCSL) (2011) *Health Cost Containment and Efficiencies* (Denver: NCSL). https://www.ncsl.org/documents/health/IntroandBriefsCC-16.pdf

National Conference of State Legislatures (NCSL) (2022) *Certificate of Need (CON) State Laws*. https://www.ncsl.org/research/health/con-certificate-of-need-state-laws.aspx

Nesi, T.J. (2008) *Poison Pills: The Untold Story of the Vioxx Scandal* (New York: Dunne).

Neville, S. (2023) Ambulance and A&E Waiting Times Hit New High in England, *Financial Times*, January 12.

Ng, T., C. Harrington and M. Kitchener (2010) Medicare and Medicaid in Long-term Care, *Health Affairs* 29, 22–28.

Nottingham, C. (2019) *The NHS in Scotland: The Legacy of the Past and the Prospect of the Future* (London: Taylor and Francis).

O'Keefe, E. (2014) The House has Voted 54 Times in Four Years on Obamacare, *Washington Post*, March 21.

Oberlander, J. (2007) Through the Looking Glass: The Politics of the Medicare Prescription Drug, Improvement and Modernization Act, *Journal of Health Politics Policy and Law* 32, 187–219.

Oberlander, J. (2018) The Republican War on Obamacare—What Has it Achieved? *New England Journal of Medicine* 379, 703–5.

Oberlander, J. and R.K. Weaver (2015) Unraveling from Within? The Affordable Care Act and Self-Undermining Policy Feedbacks, *The Forum* 13, 37–62.

Orentlicher, D. (2003) The Rise and Fall of Managed Care: A Predictable "Tragic Choices" Phenomenon, *Saint Louis University Law Journal* 47, 411–22.

Organisation for Economic Co-operation and Development (OECD) (2019) *Health Care Expenditures and Finances* (Paris: OECD).

Ortaliza, J., K. Amin and C. Cox (2022) Data Note: 2022 Medical Loss Ratio Rebates, *Kaiser Family Foundation*, June 1.

References

Ouslander, J.G. and D.C. Grabowski (2020) COVID-19 in Nursing Homes: Calming the Perfect Storm, *Journal of the American Geriatrics Society* 68, 2053–62.

Outcalt, C. (2021) "He Thought What He Was Doing Was Good For People": Why it is so Difficult to Prevent Unnecessary Medical Procedures in the U.S. Health-care Systems, *The Atlantic,* August 13.

Padget, W.R. (2003) Damage Limitations in Medical Malpractice Actions: Necessary Legislation or Unconstitutional Deprivation, *South Carolina Law Review* 55, 215–31.

Paik, M., B. Black and D. Hyman (2013) The Receding Tide of Medical Malpractice Litigation: Part 2–Effect of Damage Caps, *Journal of Empirical Legal Studies* 10, 639–69.

Pancheco-Vega, R. (2020) Environmental Regulation, Governance and Policy Instruments: 20 Years After the Stick, Carrot and Sermons Typology, *Journal of Environmental Policy & Planning* 22, 620–35.

Park, E. (2023) *Medicaid and CHIP Provisions in Biden Administration's Fiscal Year 2024 Budget* (Washington, DC: Georgetown University Health Policy Center). https://ccf.georgetown.edu/2023/03/09/medicaid-and-chip-provisions-in-biden-administrations-fiscal-year-2024-budget/

Patashnik, E. and C. Pateman (2000) *Putting Trust in the US Budget: Federal Trust Funds and the Politics of Commitment* (Cambridge: Cambridge University Press).

Patashnik, E.M., A.S. Gerber and C.M. Dowling (2017) *Unhealthy Politics: The Battle Over Evidence-based Medicine* (Princeton, NJ: Princeton University Press).

Patel, R.S., R. Bachu, A. Adikey, M. Malik and M. Shah (2018) Factors Related to Physician Burnout and its Consequences: A Review, *Behavioral Sciences* 8, October 25. https://mdpi-res.com/d_attachment/behavsci/behavsci-08-00098/article_deploy/behavsci-08-00098.pdf?version=1540460521

Pennsylvania Department of State (2022) *Disciplinary Actions of State Licensing Boards* (Harrisburg: Commonwealth of Pennsylvania).

Perez, V. and C. Wing (2019) Should We do More to Police Medicaid Fraud? Evidence on the Intended and Unintended Consequences of Expanded Enforcement, *American Journal of Health Economics* 5, 481–508.

Peter G. Peterson Foundation (PGPF) (2022) Nearly 30 Million Americans Have No Health Insurance, *Peter G. Peterson Foundation.* https://www.pgpf.org/blog/2022/11/nearly-30-million-americans-have-no-health-insurance

Peters, B.G. (2022) American Federalism in the Pandemic, in B.G. Peters, E.J. Grin and F.L. Abrucio, eds., *American Federal Systems and COVID-19* (Bingley: Emerald).

Phan-Kanter, G. (2014) Revisiting Financial Conflicts of Interest in FDA Advisory Committees, *Milbank Quarterly* 92, 446–70.

PHRMA (2022) *Patient Experience Survey, 2022* (Washington, DC: PHRMA). https://phrma.org/-/media/Project/PhRMA/PhRMA-Org/PhRMA-Refresh/Report-PDFs/P-R/PES-Report-3_RV18f.pdf

Pierre. J. and D. Carelli (2022) When the Cat is Away: How Institutional Autonomy, Low Salience and Issue Complexity Shape Administrative Behavior, Unpublished paper (Department of Political Science, University of Gothenburg).

Polsby, N.W. (1985) *Political Innovation in America: The Politics of Policy Initiation* (New Haven, CT: Yale University Press).

Pope, C. (2016) Supplemental Benefits Under Medicare Advantage, *Health Affairs*, January 21. https://www.healthaffairs.org/do/10.1377/forefront.20160121.052787

Postma, J., and A.-F. Roos (2015) Why Healthcare Providers Merge, *Health Economics, Policy and Law* 11, 121–40.

Pressman, J.L. and A. Wildavsky (1974) *Implementation* (Berkeley: University of California Press).

Rabin, D.L., A. Jetty, S. Patterson and A. Froelich (2020) Under the ACA Higher Deductibles and Medical Debt Cause Those Most Vulnerable to Defer Needed Care, *Journal of Health Care for the Poor and Underserved* 31, 424–40.

Rajkumar, S.V. (2020) The High Cost of Insulin in the United States: An Urgent Call to Action, *Mayo Clinic Proceedings* 95, 22–8.

Rau, J. (2021) Medicare Punishes 2,499 Hospitals for High Readmissions, *Kaiser Health News*, October 28.

Reed, T. (2023a) Biden's Medicare Budget May Have Some Bite, *Axios Vital Signs*, March 9. https://www.axios.com/newsletters/axios-vitals-318b2b85-5fb6-4f48-a81e-5e4e4a300494.html?chunk=0&utm_term=emshare

Reed, T. (2023b) Big Thing: State Public Option Plans Keep Hitting Obstacles, *Axios Vital Signs*, March 24. https://www.axios.com/newsletters/axios-vitals-bbdd816a-e378-4698-9284-5e515e798c38.html?chunk=0&utm_term=emshare#story0

Rettig, R.A. (1991) Origins of the Medicare Kidney Disease Entitlement: The Social Security Amendments of 1972, in K.E. Hanna, ed., *Biomedical Politics* (Washington, DC; National Academies Press).

Reverby, S.M. (2000) *Tuskegee's Truths: Rethinking the Tuskegee Syphilis Study* (Chapel Hill: University of North Carolina Press).

Robert Wood Johnson Foundation and T. H. Chan School of Public Health, Harvard University (2021) The Public's Perspective on the United States Public Health System, May. https://cdn1.sph.harvard.edu/wp-content/uploads/sites/94/2021/05/RWJF-Harvard-Report_FINAL-051321.pdf

Robinson, J.C. (2005) Health Savings Accounts—The Ownership Society in Health Care, *New England Journal of Medicine* 353, 1199–202.

Rodriguez-Rojas, A., J. Rodriguez-Beltran, A. Couce and J. Blazquez (2013) Antibiotics and Antibiotic Resistance: A Bitter Fight Against Evolution, *International Journal of Medical Microbiology* 303, 293–7.

Rosenbaum, S. and T.M. Westmoreland (2012) The Supreme Court's Surprising Decision on the Medicaid Expansion: How Will the Federal Government and the States Proceed?, *Health Affairs* 31, 85–96.

Rosenthal, E. (2017) *An American Sickness: How Healthcare Became Big Business and How You can Take it Back* (New York: Penguin).

Rosenthal, E. (2022) As Pandemic Eases Millions Could Lose Health Coverage, *New York Times*, April 6.

References

Rudowitz, R., M.B. Musumeci, R. Garfield and E. Hinton (2020) Implications of CMS's New "Healthy Adult Opportunity" Demonstrations for Medicare, *Kaiser Family Foundation.* https://www.kff.org/medicaid/issue-brief/implications-of-cmss-new-healthy-adult-opportunity-demonstrations-for-medicaid/

Russell, R.S., D.M. Johnson and S.W. White (2015) Patient Perceptions of Quality: Analyzing Patient Satisfaction Surveys, *International Journal of Operations & Production Management* 35, 1158–81.

Sachs, R. (2021) The Rhetorical Transformations and Policy Failures of Prescription Drug Pricing Reform Under the Trump Administration, *Journal of Health Politics, Policy and Law* 46, 1053–68.

Sanger-Katz, M. (2021) An 11th Hour Approval for Major Changes to Medicaid in Tennessee, *New York Times*, June 21.

Sanger-Katz, M. (2022) Build Back Better is a Health Care Bill Now, *New York Times*, July 15.

Sanger-Katz, M. (2023) The December Omnibus Bill's Little Secret: It Was Also a Giant Health Bill, *New York Times*, January 22.

Sanger-Katz, M. and S. Kliff (2021) Remember the Healthcare.gov Debacle? The Legacy Haunts the Biden Plan, *New York Times*, March 22.

Sarin, J. and Sarin, W. (2002) *Muckraking: The Journalism that Changed America* (New York: The New Press).

Schneider, S.K. (1997) Medicaid Section 1115 Waivers: Shifting Health Care Reform to the States, *Publius: The Journal of Federalism* 27, 89–109.

Schulte, F. and H.K. Hacker (2022) Hidden Audits Reveal Millions of Overcharges by Medicare Advantage Programs, *NPR*, November 21. https://www.npr.org/sections/health-shots/2022/11/21/1137500875/audit-medicare-advantage-over charged-medicare

Schwartz, L.M. and S. Wolshin (2019) Medical Marketing in the United States, 1997–2016, *JAMA Network*, January 1/8. https://jamanetwork.com/journals/jama/fullarticle/2720029

Scott, D. (2017) The Health Care Industry Doesn't Love Obamacare Enough to Save It, *Vox*, June 19. https://www.vox.com/policy-and-politics/2017/6/19/15753678/health-care-industry-lobbying-ahca

Sedhom, R. and D. Barile (2017) Teaching Our Doctors to Care for the Elderly: A Geriatric Needs Assessment Targeting Internal Medicine Residents, *Gerontology and Geriatric Medicine.* https://doi.org/10.1177%2F2333721417701687

Sekerka, L.E. and L. Benishek (2018) Thick as Thieves: Big Pharma Wields its Power with the Help of Government Regulation, *Emory Corporate Governance and Accountability Review* 5, 113–41.

Sherkow, J.S., E.Y. Adashi and L.G. Cohen (2023) Assessing—and Extending—California's Insulin Manufacturing Initiative, *JAMA Network*, January 19. https://jamanetwork.com/journals/jama/article-abstract/2800773

Shlaes, D.M. and P.A. Bradford (2018) Antibiotics—From There to Where?: How the Antibiotic Miracle is Threatened by Resistance and A Broken Market and What We Can Do About It, *Pathogens and Immunity* 3, 19–42.

Shrank, W.H., T.L. Rogstad and N. Parekh (2019) Waste in the US Health Care System: Estimated Costs and Potential for Savings, *Journal of the American Medical Association* 322, 1501–9.

Sieck, C.J., A. Sheon, J.S. Ancker, J. Castek, B. Callahan and S. Siefer (2021) Digital Inclusion as a Social Determinant of Health, *npj Digital Medicine* 4, Article 52.

Sinclair, U. (1906) *The Jungle* (New York: Doubleday).

Singh, H., T.D. Giardina, A.N.D. Meyer, S.N. Forjouh, M.D. Reis and E.J. Thomas (2013) Types and Origins of Diagnostic Errors in Primary Care Settings, *JAMA Internal Medicine* 173, 418–25.

Slaughter, L.M. (2006) Medicare Part D–The Product of a Broken Process, *New England Journal of Medicine* 354, 2314–15.

Span, P. (2022) Cancer Centers Push Testing Even to a Fault, *New York Times*, July 26.

Sparer, M.S. (2019) States as Policy Laboratories: The Politics of State-Based Single Payer Plans, *American Journal of Public Health* 109, 1511–14.

Spencer, K.L. and M. Grace (2016) Social Foundations of Health Care Inequality and Treatment Bias, *Annual Review of Sociology* 42, 101–20.

Stafford, R.S. (2012) Off-label use of Drugs and Medical Devices: A Review of Policy Implications, *Clinical Pharmacology & Therapeutics* 91, 920–5.

Starr, R.R. (2015) Too Little, Too Late: Ineffective Regulation of Dietary Supplements in the United States, *American Journal of Public Health* 105, 478–85.

Statista (2022) Direct to the Consumer Spending of the Pharmaceutical Industry in the United States from 2012 to 2021. https://www.statista.com/statistics/686 906/pharma-ad-spend-usa/

Stefanick, M.L. (2017) Doctors Must Dig into Gender Differences to Improve Women's Health Care, *Scientific American* 317, 52–7.

Stein, H.F. (2018) *American Medicine as Culture* (New York: Routledge).

Stolberg, S.G. (2022) Post-Roe, Mothers in Mississippi Get Minimal Support, *New York Times*, August 19.

Strelenhert, H., L. Richter-Sundberg, M.E. Nyström and H. Hasson (2015) Evidence-informed Policy Formulation and Implementation: A Comparative Study of two National Policies for Improving Health and Social Care in Sweden, *Implementation Science* 10, Article 169. https://implementationscience.biomedcent ral.com/articles/10.1186/s13012-015-0359-1

Studdert, D.M., M.M. Mello, and T.A. Brennan (2004) Medical Malpractice, *New England Journal of Medicine* 350, 283–92.

Sullivan, T. (2018) Defensive Practice Adds $45 Billion to the Cost of Healthcare, *Policy & Medicine,* May 5. https://www.policymed.com/2010/09/defensive-medic ine-adds-45-billion-to-the-cost-of-healthcare.html

Tankersley, J. and M. Sanger-Katz (2023) Biden Budget will Propose Tax Increase to Bolster Medicare, *New York Times*, March 7.

Taylor, J.S. (2016) What is the Real Rate of Surgical Site Infection, *Journal of Oncology Practice* 12, 878–83.

References

Thebault, R., L. Bernstein, A.B. Tran and Y. Shin (2020) Fear of Seeking Care in Hospitals Overwhelmed by the Pandemic may have Caused Thousands of Deaths, *Washington Post*, July 2.

Tracy, A. (2020) How Trump Gutted Obama's Pandemic-Preparedness Systems, *Vanity Fair*, May 1.

Tran, M. and R.K. Sokas (2017) The Gig Economy and Contingent Work: An Occupational Health Assessment, *Journal of Occupational and Environmental Medicine*, 59(4): e63–6.

Tucker, J.L. (2002) Factors Influencing Physician Participation in Medicaid in the USA, *International Journal of Social Economics* 29, 753–62.

Twenter, P. (2022) Critics Say Mark Cuban's Pharmacy Isn't Tackling the Big Issue: Brand-name Drugs, *Becker's Hospital Review*, July 28. https://www.becker shospitalreview.com/pharmacy/critics-say-mark-cuban-s-pharmacy-isn-t-tackling-the-big-issue-brand-name-drugs.html?origin=BHRE&utm_source=BHRE&utm_medium=email&utm_content=newsletter&oly_enc_id=6522 A1601390C5Z

Ullrich, F. And K. Mueller (2021) Pharmacy Vaccine Service Availability in Non-metropolitan Counties, *Rural Data Brief 2020–10*, Center for Rural Health Policy Analysis, February.

Union of Concerned Scientists (2017) Merck Manipulated the Science About the Drug Vioxx, October 12. https://www.ucsusa.org/resources/merck-manipulated-science-about-drug-vioxx

United States Government Accountability Office (USGAO) (2020) *Rural Hospital Closures* (Washington, DC: USGAO).

US Bureau of the Census (2022) Current Population Reports. https://www.census.gov/content/dam/Census/library/visualizations/2021/demo/p60-273/figure2.pdf

US Food and Drug Administration (USFDA) (2022) Prescription Drug User Fee Amendments. https://www.fda.gov/industry/fda-user-fee-programs/presription-drug-user-fee-amendmnts

Wager, E., J. Ortaliza and C. Cox (2022) How Does Health Spending in the US Compare to Other Countries?, *KFF Health Systems Tracker*, January 21.

Wallace, S.P. (2012) *Undocumented Immigrants and Healthcare Reform* (Los Angeles: UCLA Center for Health Policy Reform), August 31.

WalletHub (2022) 2022's Best and Worst States for Health Care, August 1. https://wallethub.com/edu/states-with-best-health-care/23457

Wang, A.B. (2022) Sen. Johnson Suggests Ending Medicare, Social Security as Mandatory Spending Programs, *Washington Post*, August 3.

Watson, C.R., M. Watson and T.K. Sell (2017) Public Health Preparedness Funding: Key Programs and Trends from 2001–2017, *American Journal of Public Health* 107, S165–7.

Waxman, H.A., B. Corr, J. Sharp, R. McDonald and K. Kenyatta (2020) *Getting to Lower Prescription Drug Prices* (New York: Commonwealth Fund), October.

Wennberg, J.E. (2010) *Tracking Medicine: A Researcher's Quest to Understand Healthcare* (Oxford: Oxford University Press).

Whiteman, H. (2014) 1 in 20 American Adults "Misdiagnosed in Outpatient Clinics Each Year", *Medical News Today*, April 17. https://www.medicalnewsto day.com/articles/275565

Wildavsky, A. (2018) *The Art and Craft of Policy Analysis*, rev. ed. (London: Macmillan).

Wofford, B. (2020) We're Devastatingly Short of Doctors. Why Doesn't the US Just Make More?, *The Washingtonian*, April 13.

Wolfson, B.J. (2021) Layers of Subcontracted Services Confuse and Frustrate Medi-Cal Patients, *California Healthline*, December 21.

Woolhandler, S. and D.U. Himmelstein (2013) Life or Debt: Underinsurance in America, *Journal of General Internal Medicine* 28(9): 1122–4.

Young, J.H. (1961) *The Toadstool Millionaires: A Social History of Patent Medicine in America Before Federal Regulation* (Princeton, NJ: Princeton University Press).

Zickafoose, J.S. (2020) Learning More for Children from Medicaid and CHIP Policy Experiments, *Academic Pediatrics* 20, 3–5.

Index

Index

Printed in the USA
CPSIA information can be obtained
at www.ICGtesting.com
JSHW061426060524
62622JS00010B/429